Functional Nitric Oxide Nutrition

Dietary Strategies to Prevent and Treat
Chronic Disease

Nathan S. Bryan, PhD

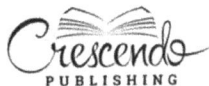

Crescendo
PUBLISHING

Functional Nitric Oxide Nutrition:
Dietary Strategies to Prevent and Treat Chronic Disease
By Nathan S. Bryan, PhD

Crescendo Publishing, LLC
2-558 Upper Gage Ave., Ste. 246
Hamilton, ON L8V 4J6
Canada

GetPublished@CrescendoPublishing.com
1-877-575-8814

ISBN: 978-1-948719-00-1 (p)

ISBN: 978-1-948719-01-8 (e)

Printed in the United States of America
Cover design by VOVO Designs

10 9 8 7 6 5 4 3 2 1

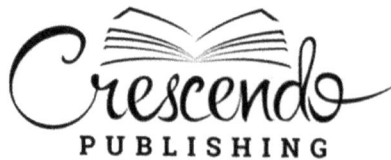

Message from the Author

Click on the link below the image to hear a special message from Dr. Bryan.

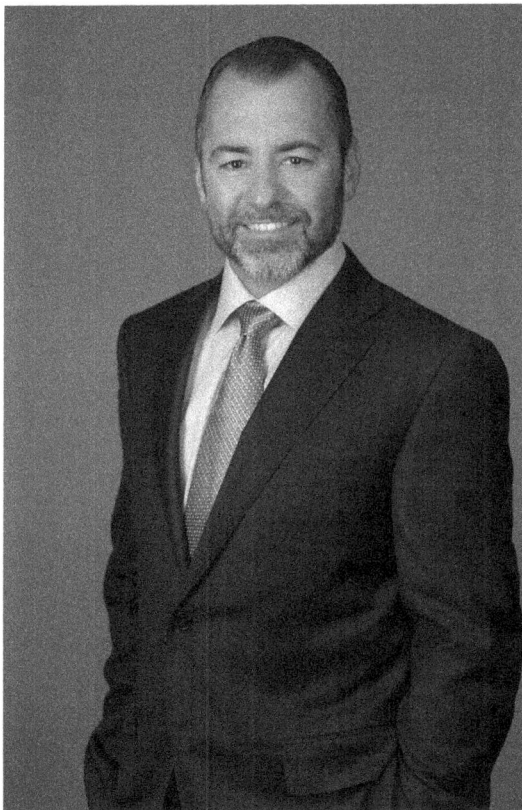

https://www.youtube.com/watch?v=LZisH_pjh7Y&t=3s

Endorsement

Dr. Nathan Bryan and I have been educating doctors at the same medical conferences for years, and have often spoken together on various aspects of nitric oxide. He explains beautifully the basics of what nitric oxide is, what it does throughout the human body to maintain health, and how it is manufactured. I have learned so much from Nathan, and his lectures always spike my interest to further my understandings and learn more about this amazing signaling gas, a gas that so few doctors know much about. Nathan truly was the original impetus to me to become an expert in nitric oxide.

As a women's health specialist, I speak on the critically important interplay between hormones, particularly estrogen and nitric oxide. Estrogen is vital to having adequate levels of nitric oxide in women. Without adequate nitric oxide, women have problems with metabolic health, blood pressure control, cognitive wellness, heart function, fertility, pregnancy, and more. There is a beautiful synergy between estrogen and nitric oxide. Without Nathan, I would not have become the well-versed physician I am with this amazing topic. All of my foundational knowledge of nitric oxide came from his teachings and research.

Dr. Bryan is a true trailblazer in this still infant field of nitric oxide, not only in researching all of the roles played by nitric oxide but also in researching the treatment of its deficiency states. He teaches the means to evaluate one's level of nitric oxide, the foundations of diet conducive to increasing nitric oxide, proper oral hygiene to allow our food to generate nitric oxide, the hazards of certain pharmaceuticals, the beneficial impact of hormones, and the role of supplementation to augment the body's production of nitric oxide.

My friend and colleague, Dr. Bryan has made a huge impact on the implementation of nitric oxide medicine to improve and even save lives. This new book he has written is a gem. I read and absorbed every word, and though I thought I would not actually learn anything new, in fact I learned quite a bit of new information from my read.

I am an integrative gynecologist and teach doctors around the world on the newest concepts in integrative women's health. All I teach on nitric oxide has evolved from my learning from Nathan. I owe him a huge debt.

There is no doubt that his new book on nitric oxide will become a groundbreaking treatise on a little appreciated and vitally important health topic. You've made a wonderful decision to buy and read this book. Enjoy it as I did, and refer back to it often. Nitric oxide should and will become an integral part of your knowledge base and approach to the care of your patients if you're a doctor. Or, it will guide your personal health choices if you're looking to optimize your own health or that of a loved one.

I celebrate the research Nathan has done in the field of nitric oxide, and I congratulate you for what you are about to do – join the world of nitric oxide literate people.

Felice Gersh, M.D.

Table of Contents

Regarding health, wouldn't it be better to build a fence at the top of a cliff than park an ambulance at the bottom?

~ Dr. Dennis Burkett

Foreword

Nitric oxide (NO) is one of the most amazing and versatile cell signaling molecules in mammalian biological systems, including cardiovascular, immunology, neurology, gastroenterology, endocrinology, pulmonary, musculoskeletal, and others. The cardiovascular effects of NO are vasodilatation, reduction in blood pressure, decrease in oxidative stress and inflammation, reduction of vascular and cardiac smooth muscle growth, inhibition of platelet aggregation, and leukocyte adhesion to the endothelium, which decreases atherosclerosis and coronary heart disease. Deficiencies of NO bioavailability are related to hypertension, atherosclerosis, coronary heart disease, both obstructive and vasospastic diabetes mellitus, dyslipidemia, and stroke. In fact, NO addresses the three finite responses to cardiovascular disease: inflammation, oxidative stress, and vascular immune dysfunction.

Numerous blood tests and noninvasive cardiovascular tests—such as asymmetric dimethyl arginine (ADMA) and devices that measure endothelial function, respectively—can access the bioavailability of NO, which is highly correlated with endothelial dysfunction, the earliest predictor of future cardiovascular events. NO also relates to arterial compliance and elasticity, which predict future coronary heart disease (CHD), stroke, and large and small arterial vascular wall disease. This can be measured with computerized arterial pulse wave analysis (CAPWA). Therefore, it is important to provide adequate NO production via the eNOS/ arginine pathway as well as the oral cavity of commensal organisms. Normal stomach acid production and symbiosis that we have with our oral microbiome provide the pathway for NO from fruits and vegetables—especially dark green leafy vegetables and beets—to convert nitrates to nitrites and then to NO. This later pathway is most important in patients after the age of 40 years.

This new data has huge implications to developing treatment strategies to lower heart disease and other modern diseases associated with NO deficiency. The ability of the Mediterranean and DASH diets (Dietary Approaches to Stop Hypertension) to reduce CHD, diabetes mellitus, lower glucose, improve lipids, and increase longevity are due to the high concentration of nitrates in the food that are converted to nitrites and NO by this system, the basis for functional nitric oxide nutrition.

Dr. Bryan has performed a masterpiece of literary genius in his new book, "Functional Nitric Oxide Nutrition." The discovery of nitric oxide production in humans is considered one of the most important medical discoveries of the last 100 years. This book will take the reader on a simple and clear journey of how to understand and use nitric oxide to maintain health and longevity. The text takes us from basic science to clinical work and therapeutics. Each chapter is well organized, and the flow from one concept to the next is smooth and effortless for the reader. Few books transform complexity to singular clarity as this one does. I recommend this excellent book to all my patients and to medical professionals who wish to enter into an education of nitric oxide from one of the leading experts and innovators in this area.

Mark C. Houston MD MS MSc FACP FAHA FASH FACN FAARM ABAARM, ABCCH.
Associate Clinical Professor of Medicine
Vanderbilt University Medical School
Director, Hypertension Institute and Vascular Biology
Medical Director of Division of Human Nutrition
Saint Thomas Medical Group, Saint Thomas Hospital
Nashville, Tennessee

Introduction

Health care and medicine have been and continue to be major issues in the U.S. The U.S. spends more money on health care than any other nation, yet we rank last or close to last for all major developed countries. These statistics are staggering, considering we know a lot about the mechanisms of disease. Scientific and medical discoveries in the past 100 years have led to enormous advancements in medical care here in the U.S. and worldwide. Primarily through vaccines and antibiotics/antiseptics, the burden of death from infectious disease has drastically declined. The advent of medical devices and advancements in emergency medicine has led to better care of trauma patients and life-threatening emergencies from acute injury. Innovations in imaging and diagnostics have led to early detection of many chronic diseases.

However, the development of safe and effective treatments or cures of chronic diseases such as cardiovascular disease, Alzheimer's disease, cancer, and diabetes have been disappointingly slow and largely ineffective. According to the 2010 National Center for Health Statistics Report, life expectancy has increased 1.1 years over the past decade, going from 76.8 to 77.9. All causes of death adjusted for age decreased by 12.5 percent from 2000 to 2008. But the percent of the population 18 years and over with heart disease has risen from 10.9 percent to 11.8 percent, and the population 65 years and over has risen from 29.6 percent to 31.7 percent over the same eight years. Diabetes has gone from 8.5 percent of the population 20 years and older to 11.9 percent in just eight years. The percentage of people with hypertension has risen from 28.9 percent to 32.6 percent. Cancer has followed a similar trend, increasing from 4.9 percent to 6.1 percent in patients 18 years old and over.

These statistics suggest that although people are living longer, they are not living better—or they are living with a chronic disease that requires care and treatment. It is the care and treatment of these chronic patients that causes the enormous economic burden on the health care system and the patients. In fact, from 2000 to 2008, total health care expenditures increased from $1.1 to $2.0 trillion, or from $4,032 to $6,411 per capita, and today a decade later are over $10,000 per capita. This highlights a very serious problem with our health care system and clearly demonstrates that what we are doing is not working. As Albert Einstein once said, "Insanity is doing the same thing over and over and expecting different results." We can, and must, do better.

The top ten causes of death in the U.S. are heart disease, cancer, chronic respiratory diseases, accidents/drugs misuse and abuse, stroke, Alzheimer's, diabetes, influenza/pneumonia, kidney disease, and suicide. Eight out of these top ten causes of death have a clear and indisputable mechanism involving nitric oxide production. I am trained in biochemistry and molecular and cellular physiology. I take great pride and responsibility in the fact that I understand how the body works and what goes wrong in people who get disease. What we have learned in nitric oxide biochemistry and physiology over the past twenty years allows us to very safely and effectively restore nitric oxide production. At the time this book was written, there are over 150,000 published scientific and medical papers on nitric oxide revealing that if you can prevent loss of nitric oxide production and availability, you can prevent many age-related chronic diseases—including 80 percent of the top ten causes of death.

The intentions of this book are to highlight new science that is not considered, or even known, by most physicians and healthcare practitioners, so patients and consumers can use this information and new knowledge to take control of their own health. My objectives are to educate readers on the importance of nitric oxide, to clearly illustrate that diet and lifestyle modifications can significantly improve nitric oxide production, and to arm the reader with information they can begin to implement into their daily life. My hope is that people will not only be able to improve their current health conditions, but prevent many of these diseases in the first place. After reading this book, I want everyone to walk away with these basic learnings:

1. Nitric oxide is one of the most important molecules produced in the human body. It controls and regulates most cellular functions.

2. Loss of nitric oxide is the earliest event in the onset and progression of most, if not all, chronic diseases.

3. As we age, we lose the ability to produce nitric oxide, putting us at risk for age-related diseases.

4. New discoveries in science and medicine reveal what goes wrong in people who can't make nitric oxide. We now know how to fix these basic problems with simple diet and lifestyle changes, without drug intervention.

With these four basic concepts and by employing the strategies I teach you in this book, you can make great progress to improve your current health status, whether you are sick and hoping to get better or currently healthy and just want to prevent getting sick.

This book is organized to provide a historical account of discoveries in nutrition so you can become aware that what I am describing is not dissimilar to transformative health and disease discoveries that occurred many years ago. I then want to introduce the concept of how nitric oxide (NO) is produced from nitrate and nitrite found in many of the foods we eat. This will provide the background for why functional nutrition focused on NO will transform public health. The next few chapters provide some complicated steps and pathways that are necessary and sufficient for adequate NO production. The role of bacteria is essential.

Next, I describe why vegetables are good for you. It goes beyond simple antioxidants and the vitamins and minerals they provide. Historically, we have been misinformed that nitrite and nitrate are toxic food additives only found in hot dogs and bacon. I will properly inform you on the true science around nitrite and nitrate, and provide perspective on the major sources of nitrite and nitrate in our diet. The following chapters review the published scientific literature on how much we need to get in our diet to achieve the clinical benefits of consuming such amounts. The final chapters provide a clear program and guidelines for what you can do to make sure your NO levels remain adequate to support your own physiology, whether you are a young, well-trained athlete or a senior citizen wanting to improve your quality of life. Finally, I will provide my perspective on where NO science may take us in the future.

The field of nitric oxide is relatively new. The molecule was only discovered in the late 1970s and early 1980s. In fact, it is one of the newest discoveries in medicine. Very few people, including physicians treating patients, know about nitric oxide. My hope is that through this book and others, nitric oxide will become as well-known as omega-3 fatty acids or vitamin C. The science is clear that without sufficient nitric oxide production, your body cannot and will not heal, nor will it perform optimally. The single most important thing you can do for your health is to improve or restore normal nitric oxide production. This book will help you do just that.

- 1 -

History of Nutrition

Advancements in nutrition and discoveries of new nutrients have had revolutionary effects on health and disease management throughout history. The word nutrition itself means the process of nourishing or being nourished, especially the process by which a living organism assimilates food and uses it for growth and replacement of tissues. A nutrient is defined as any substance that nourishes an organism, and to nourish is to sustain with food or nutriment—to supply with what is necessary for life, health, and growth. Nutrients, therefore, are substances that are essential to life that must be supplied by food. Some categories of nutrients include water, protein, carbohydrates, vitamins, minerals, fatty acids, and amino acids. There are obviously many specific examples within each of the categories. What is clear, though, is that nutrients are fundamental to physiological systems, and good nutrition can prevent many diseases. It follows that the absence of nutrients can cause disease. We and others have recently discovered a new set of nutrients, the lack of which may be the cause of all chronic diseases—including cardiovascular disease, the number one killer of men and women worldwide. To the contrary, sufficient ingestion or supplementation of these specific nutrients may prevent many of these chronic diseases.

Today more than ever, gaining nutrition knowledge can make a transformative impact on our lives. Air, soil, and water pollution, in addition to changing farming practices, have depleted our soils of vital and essential nutrients and minerals. The widespread use of food additives, chemicals, sugar, and unhealthy fats in our diets contributes to many of the degenerative diseases of our day such as cancer, heart disease, arthritis, and osteoporosis. We know a poor diet causes many health problems such as blindness, anemia, scurvy, preterm birth, stillbirth, and cretinism. Diet and nutrient-related issues can also lead to health-threatening conditions like obesity and metabolic syndrome, and even common chronic systemic diseases as cardiovascular disease, diabetes, and osteoporosis. In order to appreciate the recent discovery of a new nutrient that is essential for optimal health, it is important to understand central historical milestones in nutrition.

In 400 B.C., Hippocrates, the "Father of Medicine," said to his students, "Let thy food be thy medicine and thy medicine be thy food." Isn't it ironic that we have abandoned food and nutrition as a staple of modern medicine? In fact, although 25 hours of nutrition instruction is recommended in the medical school curriculum, many physicians report having enough nutrition knowledge to counsel and treat their patients. Perhaps it is time to get back to the basics, especially when modern medicine fails us miserably today. This is apparent in the U.S., which has been ranked as one of the lowest developed countries in health care despite spending more than any other country.

In the same era as Hippocrates in 400 B.C., foods were often used as cosmetics or medicines for the treatment of wounds. In some of the early Far Eastern biblical writings, there were references to food and health. One story describes the treatment of eye disease, now known to be due to a vitamin A deficiency, by squeezing the juice of liver onto the eye. Vitamin A is now known to be stored in large amounts in the liver, so this is the basis for the successful treatment.

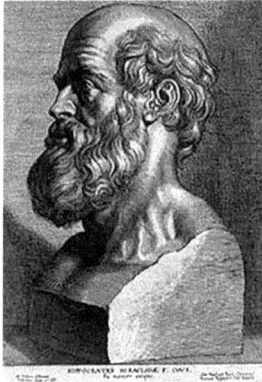

"Let food be thy medicine and medicine be thy food" – Hippocrates

PALEOSPIRIT.COM

During the 1500s, scientist and artist Leonardo da Vinci compared the process of metabolism in the body to the burning of a candle. This revealed that he had at least a conceptual understanding of how our body utilizes nutrients to fuel energy production. In 1747, Dr. James Lind, a physician in the British Navy, performed the first scientific experiment in nutrition. At that time, sailors were sent on long voyages for years and they developed scurvy (a painful, deadly, bleeding disorder). During this time, only nonperishable food products such as dried meat and breads were taken on the voyages, since there was no refrigeration and fresh foods would spoil. In his experiment to try and figure out how to treat these sailors, Lind gave some of the sailors sea water, others vinegar, and the rest limes. Only those given the limes were saved from scurvy. We now know that the vitamin C in the limes is what prevented the scurvy. However, vitamin C wasn't discovered until the 1930s, or almost 200 years after Lind's experiment.

Lind didn't know it at the time, but he had discovered a vital nutrient.

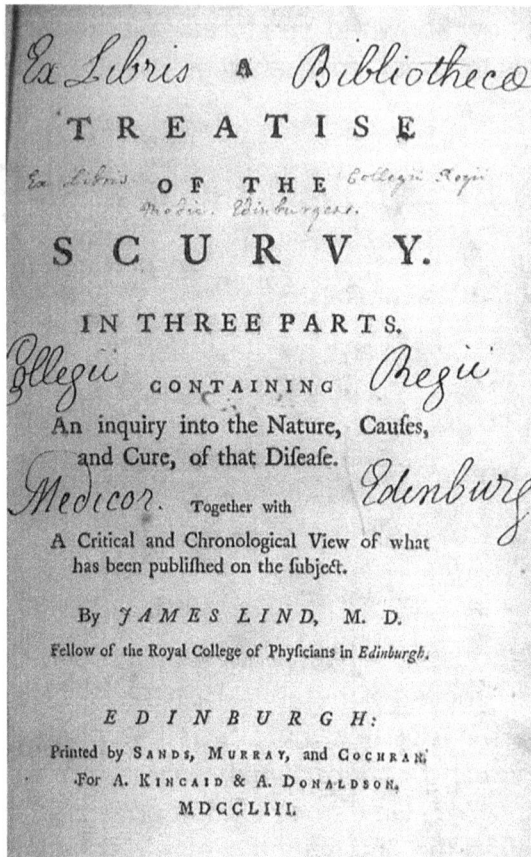

In 1790, George Fordyce recognized calcium as necessary for fowl survival. In the early 1800s, it was discovered that foods are composed primarily of four elements—carbon, nitrogen, hydrogen, and oxygen—and methods were developed for determining the amounts of these elements. Justus Liebig of Germany, a pioneer in early plant growth studies, was the first to point out the chemical makeup of carbohydrates, fats, and proteins. Carbohydrates were made of sugars, fats were fatty acids, and proteins were made up of amino acids. Just before the turn of the 20th century, in 1897, Christiaan Eijkman, a Dutchman working with natives in Java, observed that some of the natives developed a disease called beriberi, which caused heart problems and paralysis. He recognized that chickens, when fed the native diet of white rice, also developed the symptoms of beriberi. When he fed the chickens unprocessed brown rice (with the outer bran intact), they did not develop the disease. Based on his observations in chickens, Eijkman then fed brown rice to his patients and they were cured of beriberi. This was another important case demonstrating that specific nutrients found in certain foods could cure disease. Nutritionists later learned that the outer rice bran contains vitamin B1, also known as thiamine, a deficiency of which is the cause of beriberi.

In the early 1900s, E.V. McCollum, while working for the U.S. Department of Agriculture at the University of Wisconsin, developed an approach that opened the way to the widespread discovery of nutrients. He discovered the first fat soluble vitamin, vitamin A. He found that rats fed butter were healthier than those fed lard, as butter contains more vitamin A. About the same time, Dr. Casmir Funk was the first to coin the term "vitamins" as vital factors in the diet. He wrote about these unidentified substances present in food, which could prevent the diseases of scurvy, beriberi, and pellagra (a disease caused by a deficiency of niacin, vitamin B-3). The term vitamin is derived from the words vital and amine, because vitamins are required for life and they were originally thought to be amines—nitrogen compounds derived from ammonia. We will discuss nitrogen based nutrients in subsequent chapters.

In 1925, E.B. Hart discovered that trace amounts of copper are necessary for iron absorption. In 1927, Adolf Otto Reinhold Windaus synthesized vitamin D, for which he won the Nobel Prize in Chemistry in 1928. In 1928, Albert Szent-Györgyi isolated ascorbic acid, and in 1932 proved that vitamin C prevented scurvy. In 1935, he synthesized it, and in 1937, he won a Nobel Prize for his efforts. In the 1930s, William Rose discovered the essential amino acids, the building blocks of protein.

In 1968, Linus Pauling, a Nobel Prize winner in chemistry, created the term orthomolecular nutrition. Orthomolecular is, literally, "pertaining to the right molecule." Pauling proposed that by giving the body the right molecules in the right concentration (optimum nutrition), people could use nutrients to achieve better health and prolong life. There is substantial scientific and clinical evidence to support that the right nutrients are found in the right concentrations in whole foods (when grown in nutrient dense soils). Therefore, consuming a balance of the right foods containing different essential nutrients and vitamins should be able to prevent and/or treat/ cure many diseases. Pauling himself said that most diseases are caused by nutrient deficiencies.

My research program was the first to demonstrate the absence of nitrite and nitrate in the diet made many disease conditions worsen, including injury from heart attack. We were also the first to demonstrate that supplementing or restoring these missing nutrients back into the diet, reversed the disease and injury and could actually prevent chronic inflammation (main driver of disease). These were some of the first discoveries in this era of "functional nitric oxide nutrition".

These discoveries over the years have led many scientists and pharmaceutical companies to begin to isolate active compounds from foods and synthesize them to sell as vitamins or dietary supplements, or create derivatives they could then patent. It is clear from history that these active compounds can cure, treat, and even prevent disease. The timeline below chronologically illustrates how these discoveries have led to amelioration of many diseases and the beginning of the functional nitric oxide nutrition era. The following chapters will highlight how these handful of discoveries have the potential to change the face of medicine and health care. Simply restoring functional nutrients that are missing in much of the population and certainly missing in sick people can restore cellular function and improve human health. History has a pattern of repeating itself and has demonstrated unequivocally that giving back a missing nutrient has profound effects on human health and disease.

If that's the case, if nutrients really do have impact on human health and disease, you might be wondering why vitamins, nutrients, and supplement packaging labels include a phrase saying that their products and information are not intended to diagnose, treat, cure, or prevent any disease. These also usually state that their health claims have not been evaluated by the Food and Drug Administration (FDA). In October of 1994, the U.S. Congress passed the Dietary and Supplement Health and Education Act (DSHEA). It sets forth what can and cannot be said about nutritional supplements without prior FDA review. Many believe this is advocated by large pharmaceutical companies to protect their "drugs" for the treatment of disease. If drug companies have competition from vitamins or supplements, then this will obviously affect their profits. In January of 2000, the FDA clarified that supplement makers can state their products can improve the structure or function of the body or improve common, minor symptoms. Examples of allowable statements include "maintains a healthy heart," "helps you relax," supports healthy digestion," "is good for symptoms of PMS," "strengthens joint structure," etc. Overall, due to this law, vitamin, herb, and nutrient manufacturers have greater freedom to say what their products can do to improve our health.

While this law limits what vitamin manufacturers can claim about preventing or curing diseases, its passage has been a major milestone in the natural health field. It acknowledges the millions of people who believe dietary supplements can improve their diets and bestow good health. It opens the way for people to obtain the information they need to make the best nutritional choices. It is also very important for there to be some safety and oversight on nutritional supplements and vitamins so consumers can be certain they are actually taking and getting what the product label indicates.

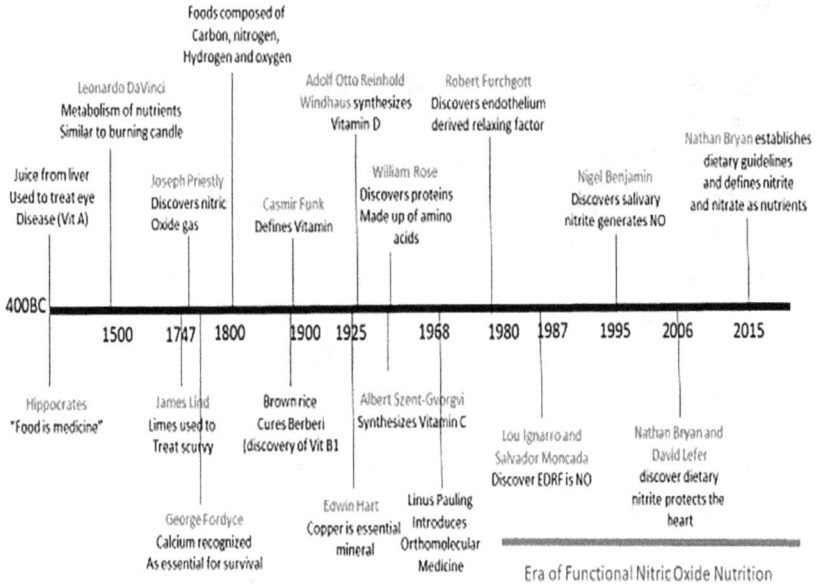

Foods composed of Carbon, nitrogen, Hydrogen and oxygen

Leonardo DaVinci
Metabolism of nutrients
Similar to burning candle

Adolf Otto Reinhold Windhaus synthesizes Vitamin D

Robert Furchgott
Discovers endothelium derived relaxing factor

Nathan Bryan establishes dietary guidelines and defines nitrite and nitrate as nutrients

Juice from liver
Used to treat eye
Disease (Vit A)

Joseph Priestly
Discovers nitric
Oxide gas

Casmir Funk
Defines Vitamin

William Rose
Discovers proteins
Made up of amino acids

Nigel Benjamin
Discovers salivary
nitrite generates NO

400BC | 1500 | 1747 | 1800 | 1900 | 1925 | 1968 | 1980 | 1987 | 1995 | 2006 | 2015

Hippocrates
"Food is medicine"

James Lind
Limes used to
Treat scurvy

Brown rice
Cures Berberi
(discovery of Vit B)

Albert Szent-Gyorgyi
Synthesizes Vitamin C

Lou Ignarro and
Salvador Moncada
Discover EDRF is NO

Nathan Bryan and
David Lefer
discover dietary
nitrite protects the
heart

George Fordyce
Calcium recognized
As essential for survival

Edwin Hart
Copper is essential
mineral

Linus Pauling
Introduces
Orthomolecular
Medicine

Era of Functional Nitric Oxide Nutrition

Understanding how nutrients and active molecules have been discovered from foods even thousands of years ago—before we had any of the advanced technology and analytical tools we have today—provides a strong foundation for the next chapters. Moving forward, we'll uncover a very important, newly discovered nutrient that may be able to cure, prevent, and treat the number one killer of men and women worldwide: cardiovascular disease. This new nutrient may very well be the most important nutrient ever discovered. Imagine a nutrient that could prevent heart disease, Alzheimer's, diabetes, and chronic infections. Keep reading, because the next chapters will not only describe this nutrient, but also provide the robust scientific evidence that it can indeed prevent, treat, or cure all of the above.

- 2 -

What is Nitric Oxide and How is it Produced?

Imagine, for a moment, a single molecule that can dramatically improve your health—and you can maintain normal levels of it within your body simply through diet and lifestyle. This single molecule can: prevent high blood pressure (hypertension); combat a disease that damages your heart, brain, and kidneys; keep your arteries young and flexible; prevent, slow, or reverse the buildup of artery-clogging arterial plaques; help stop the formation of artery-clogging blood clots (the result of plaques bursting and spilling their contents into the blood stream); and lower triglycerides. By doing all of the above, this molecule can also reduce your risk of heart attack and stroke—the first and fifth killers of men and women worldwide.

That in itself would be pretty remarkable, but this molecule can additionally reduce the risk of diabetes and disastrous diabetic complications such as chronic kidney disease, blindness, hard-to-heal foot and leg ulcers, and amputations. It also has the ability to limit the swelling and pain of arthritis, boost the power of pain-relieving drugs, reverse erectile dysfunction (ED), calm the choking inflammation of asthma, protect your bones from osteoporosis, help provide the mood-lifting power behind antidepressant medications, assist the immune system in killing bacteria, and limit skin damage from the sun.

A lack or deficiency of this molecule is what causes most diseases, including cardiovascular disease, the number one killer of men and women worldwide. That is why the scientific and medical community is so excited that this molecule can be restored and optimized through nutrition from specific foods and diet. As 1998 Nobel Laureate Louis J. Ignarro, Ph.D., said: "There may be no disease process where this miracle molecule does not have a protective role."

You can stop imagining this miracle molecule now, because it's real and accessible. What is it? Nitric oxide—otherwise known (by its chemical formula) as NO.

What is nitric oxide? It is a signaling molecule. In fact, it is how cells in our body communicate with one another. Nitric oxide is NO, one atom of nitrogen and one atom of oxygen—simple as can be. So simple, in fact, that it's a gas when it is produced within the body. When it's created and released by cells, this gas easily and quickly penetrates nearby membranes and other cells, sending its signals. In less than a second, NO signals:

- arteries to relax and expand
- immune cells to kill bacteria and cancer cells
- brain cells to communicate with each other

In fact, NO sends crucial signals within every cell, tissue, organ, and system of the body. This all occurs when our body produces nitric oxide upon demand. We now know that there are two pathways to make NO in the human body.

The endothelial cells

These are cells that line all our blood vessels throughout the circulatory system, and they generate NO from L-arginine. In young, healthy blood vessels, this pathway is functional and generates sufficient NO to maintain normal blood pressure and the integrity of the circulatory system.

Dietary nitrate and nitrite consumption

Nitrate is found primarily in green leafy vegetables and root vegetables. It is broken down into nitrite and nitric oxide based on bacteria that live in and on our body.

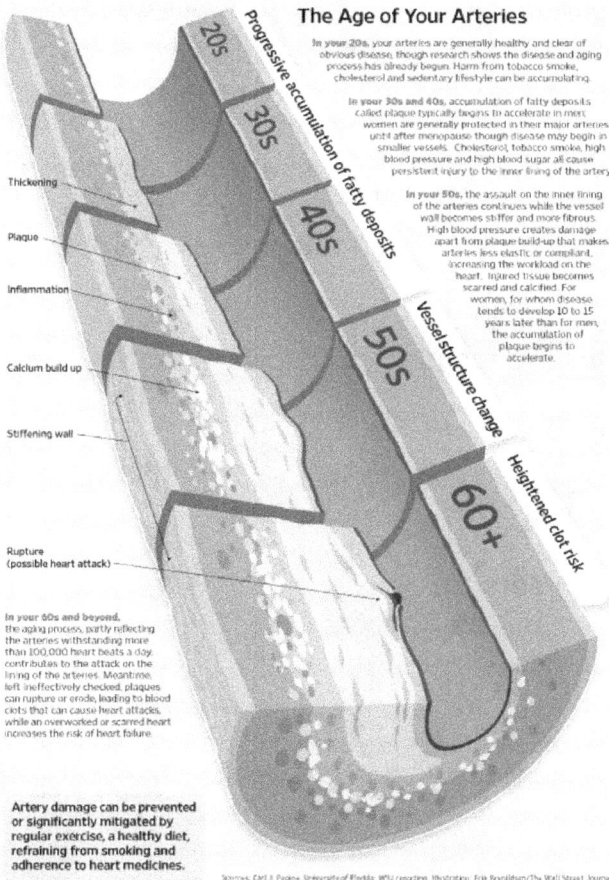

The Age of Your Arteries

In your 20s, your arteries are generally healthy and clear of obvious disease, though research shows the disease and aging process has already begun. Harm from tobacco smoke, cholesterol and sedentary lifestyle can be accumulating.

In your 30s and 40s, accumulation of fatty deposits called plaque typically begins to accelerate in men; women are generally protected in their major arteries until after menopause though disease may begin in smaller vessels. Cholesterol, tobacco smoke, high blood pressure and high blood sugar all cause persistent injury to the inner lining of the artery.

In your 50s, the assault on the inner lining of the arteries continues while the vessel wall becomes stiffer and more fibrous. High blood pressure creates damage apart from plaque build-up that makes arteries less elastic or compliant, increasing the workload on the heart. Injured tissue becomes scarred and calcified. For women, for whom disease tends to develop 10 to 15 years later than for men, the accumulation of plaque begins to accelerate.

In your 60s and beyond, the aging process, partly reflecting the arteries withstanding more than 100,000 heart beats a day, contributes to the attack on the lining of the arteries. Meantime, left ineffectively checked, plaques can rupture or erode, leading to blood clots that can cause heart attacks, while an overworked or scarred heart increases the risk of heart failure.

Artery damage can be prevented or significantly mitigated by regular exercise, a healthy diet, refraining from smoking and adherence to heart medicines.

The endothelial pathway (pathway 1) becomes disrupted with age. There are conditions where either one or both pathways become disrupted. If one system goes down, the other one can compensate and pull the weight for the other. However, if both systems fail, then you are in trouble and disease will start to set in. The older you are, the lower your NO, because of the age-related decline in endothelial function. We lose about 10 to 12 percent of our endothelial-produced NO per decade. In fact, by the time we are about 40 years old, we have lost about 50 percent of our ability to generate NO from our endothelial cells.

In one study, Italian researchers evaluated forearm blood flow—the standard measurement of endothelial health—in 47 people with normal blood pressure and 49 people with high blood pressure. They found that in both groups, those who were older had poorer endothelial-dependent vasodilation— the NO-sparked ability of arteries to widen and permit health-giving blood flow. That weakening of the endothelium was in perfect parallel to aging; decade by decade, NO-powered, endothelial-dependent vasodilation declined. Specifically:

- **30 years old and younger**
  Endothelial-dependent vasodilation was strongest.

- **31 to 45 years old**
  Vasodilation was 11 percent weaker than in the 30-and-younger set.

- **46 to 60 years old**
  Vasodilation was 13 percent weaker than in the 31 to 45-year-olds.

- **60 and older**
  Vasodilation was 28 percent weaker than in the 46- to 60-year-olds.

All in all, those 60 and older had vasodilation that was 52 percent weaker—less than half as strong—as those 30 and younger. And these were older people who did not have high blood pressure. Having high blood pressure actually accelerates this entire process. Therefore, effectively managing your blood pressure is the single most important thing you can do to protect your blood vessels and the function of all organs, tissues, and cells.

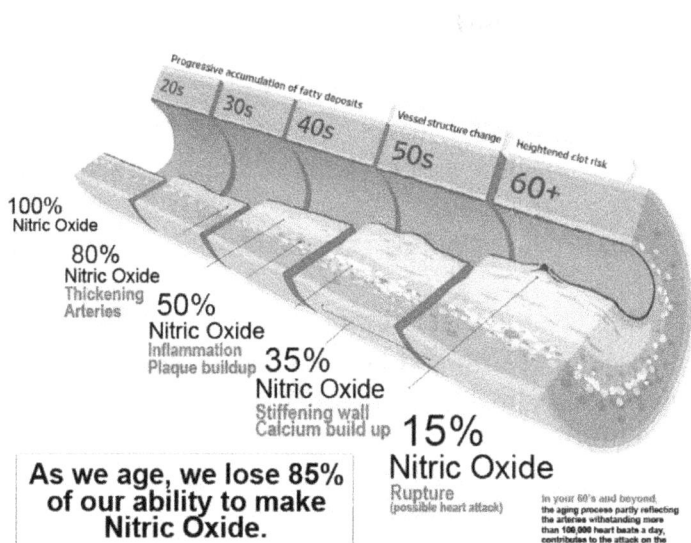

"Advancing age is an independent factor leading to the progressive impairment of endothelium-dependent vasodilation in humans," conclude researchers in the Science journal Circulation, which is published by the American Heart Association. The functional changes in the endothelium precede the structural changes seen in vascular disease by many years, sometimes decades. But why do blood vessels become dysfunctional with age?

According to the researchers, dysfunction occurs because of "A progressive reduction of NO availability." In fact, their findings suggest that "in aged individuals NO availability is almost totally compromised." In a similar study, Japanese researchers tested vasodilation in 18 healthy people, aged 23 to 70. The patients' responses to the vasodilator is striking, showing a near-perfect correlation between age and endothelial health. A 23-year-old in the study had an artery that expanded more than five times its width when given a vasodilator. The artery of the 70-year-old expanded a little more than two times. The researchers concluded: "Coronary blood flow response to acetylcholine (an endothelium-dependent vasodilator) decreased significantly with aging."

Why? Because of the age-related decrease in the release of "endothelium-derived relaxing factor or NO." Specifically, another study by the same team of Japanese researchers found a loss of 75 percent of endothelium-produced NO in people 70 to 80 years old as compared to 20-year-olds.

It's important to emphasize that this decline happens not only to people with CVD, but in healthy older adults too. These are people who don't have high blood pressure, high cholesterol, or circulation-damaging diabetes. In other words, it happens to everybody who gets older. It follows that if NO is so critical for optimal health and disease prevention, if we could figure out how to prevent the decline in NO production with aging, then perhaps we could prevent many age-related diseases. This would truly be the "holy grail" in cardiovascular medicine.

With more than 150,000 papers published on NO, the scientific and medical literature tells us that loss of NO production and availability is the earliest event in the onset and progression of cardiovascular disease. In fact, this molecule is so important that the scientists who discovered it were awarded a Nobel Prize in Medicine or Physiology in 1998. Years prior in 1992, NO was proclaimed "Molecule of the Year" by Science Magazine. Dr. Valentin Fuster, the former President of the American Heart Association and the head of cardiology at Mount Sinai Hospital in Manhattan, says that "the discovery of nitric oxide and its function is one of the most important in the history of cardiovascular medicine."

NO does more than just regulate our cardiovascular system. Our immune system is very intimately related to NO production. During the past two decades, NO has been recognized as one of the most versatile players in the immune system. It is involved in the pathogenesis and control of infectious diseases, tumors, autoimmune processes and chronic degenerative diseases. To regulate immune responses, NO will kill off invading pathogens from bacteria, to viruses on the one hand and on the other hand modulate immunosuppression during tissue-restoration and wound-healing processes. Much of these effects comes from the effects NO has upon immune cells.

NO is also important in stem cells. Mesenchymal stem cells are immune modulators. They will help suppress the inflammatory response that the body produces in many different conditions. Nitric oxide works hand in hand with mesenchymal stem cells and macrophages to make the stem cell environment more conducive for stem cell repair. There is essentially no pathological condition in the body where NO does not play a role in the management of the condition. This is another example of how losing the ability to make NO will hinder your body's ability to heal and fight off infections.

Since NO production becomes compromised with aging, older people must then rely on consuming nitrate in their diet to achieve an optimal level of NO in their system. Under ideal conditions, both pathways—endothelial production and dietary NO consumptions—provide about 50 percent of our total body NO. Thus, when both are working and functioning properly, we make sufficient NO and all the systems in our body are functioning properly. Scientific research has figured out how to "fix" the problem of lost NO from pathway 1 with age, and it has discovered how to optimize pathway 2 so that no matter how old people get, they can still have sufficient NO production to become resistant to disease.

Since NO is a gas that is gone in less than a second after it is produced within the body, it is not simple to supplement the body with NO gas. Therefore, an understanding of how the body makes NO is required, so we can then provide the body with the raw material and nutrients it needs to efficiently produce NO. Nutrients, remember, are substances that are essential to life and must be supplied by food. Since NO itself cannot be delivered in foods, we must identify the precursors (i.e. the building blocks) of this molecule that become the nutrients necessary for NO production: nitrite and nitrate.

What we now know about NO may explain a very early concept around what "animates" humans. The Roman physician Galen based his description of the vascular system on the concept of "pneuma," or spirits—a vital principle consisting of matter in a finely divided or ethereal state that flowed through the vascular and nervous systems and animated the entire organism. Many diseases were thought to owe their origin to some disturbances of these ethereal spirits. This paradigm actually prevented the advancement of medical science for centuries. But today, evidence on the production and effects of such an ethereal substance, NO, does exist. Nitric oxide is indeed formed in many organs and has important roles in physiology and pathophysiology.

Even earlier in Ancient Chinese medicine and culture, the concept of Qi (pronounced chi) was introduced. "Qi" (氣) literally means gas in Chinese. Chinese medicine has long recognized that gasses in the body have important functions such as: warming, energizing, and communicating with metabolic functions (See table below). Medically, there are names for many kinds of gasses based on their actions in the body. While they lacked the technology to identify and measure the exact gasses, Chinese physicians were keenly aware of how these gasses permeated the body and the points at which they exited the skin. Nitric oxide has been suggested to be Qi. It can pass freely through membranes, and transmit signals from neurons to target cells. When NO is out of balance, bad things typically happen. Nitric oxide has well-defined functions. It sends messages to tell cells how much energy they should be producing. When the right proportion of NO reaches fat stores, they begin to transform fat into useable energy and heat.

Comparison of Qi and Nitric Oxide

Qi	Nitric Oxide
Can travel through the body.	Can travel through the body.
Provides a communication function in the body with many metabolic reactions and processes.	Provides a communication function in the body with many metabolic reactions and processes.
Is created by combining breath and food.	NO is created from food and the cells along the sinuses and airways from a combination of gasses drawn in from the lungs, amino acids, and endogenous production from microbiota. NO can be synthesized from most cells types.
Is influenced by a special gas in the kidneys, which is associated with sexual function.	NO is the molecule that dilates blood vessels and is responsible for sexual function.
Serves as a source of energy.	Mitochondria release nitric oxide, which signals the breakdown of fat into usable energy and tells mitochondria to begin producing more ATP. ATP is the body's energy currency.
When Qi is unevenly distributed, it causes a lack of energy.	Nitric oxide regulates metabolism of energy. However, high concentrations of nitric oxide inhibit mitochondrial respiration and limit energy production.
Has a warming function.	NO converts fat into heat. It can improve the thermogenesis of brown fat.
Involved with the body's metabolism.	Involved with the body's metabolism.
Has overlapping functions with nerves, but cannot be limited to nerves alone.	Nerves release NO, which travels through membranes and makes its way to other nerves.

Controls blood circulation and has a close relationship with blood.	Nitric oxide dilates blood vessels, influencing blood circulation.
Travels along acupuncture channels.	NO is higher at acupoints/meridians and exits at acupuncture points.
Too much causes inflammation. This is known as "liver Qi stagnation."	High levels of NO are toxic and cause inflammation (oxidative damage to the liver).
Influences water metabolism.	NO plays an important role in controlling enzymes such as sodium potassium ATPase. This enzyme is essential for the body's cellular pumps to control how much water is kept inside cells.
Can be directed by intention.	Neurotransmitters release nitric oxide.
Facilitates the actions of the internal organs and endocrine system.	Facilitates the actions of the internal organs and endocrine system.
Its even flow influences emotional states and endocrine function.	Herbal formulas that have a sedative influence on the body seem to lower levels of nitric oxide. In addition, acupuncture therapy—which is used to regulate the flow of nitric oxide in the body—has been shown to be effective for depression.
Controls gut balance.	NO kills off certain microorganisms while allowing others to thrive. Oral and gut bacteria actually produce NO to maintain intestinal health.

Fundamental medical and physiological properties of molecules described centuries ago are consistent with what we know today about NO. We now have a firm understanding and convergence of many ancient and effective medical strategies that revolve around NO. We now know that we can improve the production of this molecule from foods and nutrients that many people are missing. It appears that we may have identified a critical component of our diet that many people are missing. In fact, certain things we have been taught to fear and avoid in our diet may be saving our lives from inflammatory diseases.

- 3 -

How is Nitric Oxide Derived from Nutrients?

Have you ever wondered why salads are served before the main course? Natural social behaviors, although we don't always think about it, exist for biochemical and physiological reasons. If they didn't, they would work themselves out of societal behavior. Since the late 1970s, we knew that dietary nitrate found primarily in green leafy vegetables (salads) would be absorbed in our gut and then recirculated and concentrated in our salivary glands. At that time, it was not known why our bodies would do this—especially since at that time nitrate was considered a precursor to nitrosamines that could cause cancer. Well, advance the science forty years and we now have a clear understanding of why nitrate from green leafy vegetables is absorbed and concentrated in our saliva. It is nature's way of protecting us from post-prandial (after a meal) inflammation or the damage and oxidation caused from digesting and breaking down complex foods such as proteins, fats, and carbohydrates that happens after we digest salad prior to the meal. This occurs through a human nitrogen cycle, called the enterosalivary circulation of nitrate.

Since nitric oxide is so critical to our health and our bodies can produce it from specific nutrients in the foods we eat, nature designed an exquisite system utilizing the bacteria in our mouth (the oral microbiome) to provide a source of NO from the foods we eat. Research has shown that critically ill patients who are intubated and fed through a feeding tube do not get any nitric oxide produced from this pathway since these processes prevent saliva flow, chewing, and swallowing saliva. Furthermore, people who use mouthwash disrupt this pathway and become deficient in NO. More on this later.

Nitrate found in salad greens or most leafy green vegetables can be metabolized by certain and select bacteria that live on the back part of our tongue. When we chew and eat slowly, this allows the nutrients in the food to reach the crypts of the tongue for the bacteria to reduce (break down the nitrate molecule) to nitrite and nitric oxide. Since this first part of digestion is only occurring for a period of 10 to 20 seconds at a time, there is limited opportunity for all the nitrate to reach the bacteria. Then, when we swallow the chewed up food, it is in the stomach for several minutes (45 to 120, depending on a number of factors) where it is broken down further. Food is then emptied into the upper part of the small intestines called the duodenum. It is here where nitrate is selectively taken up across the lining of the gut and then recirculated to the salivary glands. Each time we salivate, the nitrate in our saliva is broken down to nitrite and NO.

This is illustrated below:

Dietary Nitrate and Nitrite Metabolism

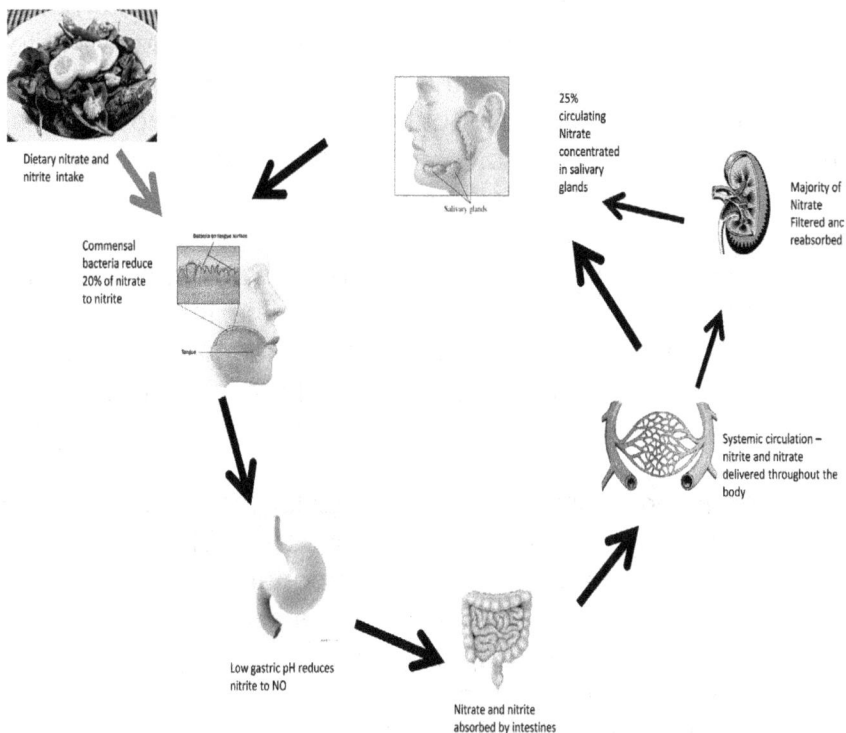

Dietary nitrate and nitrite intake

Commensal bacteria reduce 20% of nitrate to nitrite

25% circulating Nitrate concentrated in salivary glands

Salivary glands

Majority of Nitrate Filtered anc reabsorbed

Systemic circulation – nitrite and nitrate delivered throughout the body

Low gastric pH reduces nitrite to NO

Nitrate and nitrite absorbed by intestines

This process occurs slowly over the course of several hours, so that each time we salivate for the next few hours, the nitrate is utilized by bacteria that live in the crypts of the tongue as an energy source and in the process the bacteria generate nitrite. Nitrite and nitrate are distinctly different molecules, although they sound nearly the same and most people confuse them for one another. Nitrate and nitrite in the saliva are as much as 100 times higher than in the circulation. Each time we swallow our saliva, it reaches the stomach—which is very acidic—and the nitrite in saliva becomes nitric oxide gas. However, this is dependent upon sufficient stomach acid production. People who take proton pump inhibitors (Prevacid, Prilosec, etc.) for reflux disease disrupt this pathway. We will talk about this in more detail later.

The nitric oxide produced from this pathway has many beneficial functions besides dilating blood vessels internally. It is this nitric oxide gas that is generated from salivary nitrite that helps kill foodborne pathogens such as E.coli, Listeria, Chlostridium botulinum. Not only does it kill off bad bacteria that may cause sickness, but it also kills off Helicobacter pylori, the bacteria that is responsible for gastric ulcers. NO generated from swallowing our own saliva is also responsible for increasing blood flow to the stomach to help with the absorption of nutrients, and to promote the integrity of the protective lining of the stomach to prevent damage from acid. We now know how each step in this process can become disrupted and what the consequences are in specific patients.

The production of nitric oxide from swallowing our own saliva is dependent upon stomach acid production. The production of stomach acid may be the most important process for the health of all humans. The nitrite that is concentrated in our saliva from the action of nitrate-reducing bacteria becomes nitric oxide gas when the pH falls below 4. As long as the inside of the stomach is acidic, NO is generated each time we swallow. Patients taking proton pump inhibitors (PPIs or acid reflux medications) intentionally inhibit stomach acid production; therefore, the pH of the stomach is no longer acidic and no nitric oxide is produced. It is now clear that patients who have been taking PPIs for 3 to 5 years have a 30 percent higher incidence of heart attack and stroke. This is due to insufficient nitric oxide production. Can you begin to recognize the importance of NO? If its synthesis is shut down, you increase your risk of heart attack and stroke. Independent of nitric oxide production, stomach acid is required for the breakdown of proteins we consume in our diet. The enzymes in our stomach that break down protein into amino acids are only active when the stomach is acidic. When there is insufficient stomach acid production from PPI use, proteins are not broken down completely and are then undigested protein fragments (peptides) that are absorbed across our gut.

These peptides are then recognized by our immune systems as a foreign substance and this activates our immune system. This is the reason for food-borne allergies and many auto-immune diseases. With proton pump inhibitors being the third largest class of prescribed drugs worldwide, millions of people take them—generating tens of billions of dollars in revenue for pharmaceutical companies. The inhibition of nitric oxide production combined with auto-immune conditions and insufficient nutrient absorption make these drugs potentially the most dangerous drugs on the market for long-term use. However, many people become dependent upon these drugs and are unable to stop taking them. Obviously, this would be best—but for those who cannot, utilizing functional nitric oxide nutrition can partially overcome the inhibition caused by these drugs. Therefore, for those patients taking antacids, they must incorporate some form of nitric oxide nutrition that can provide a source of NO under these conditions. The last chapter will illustrate how to do just that.

In order to understand what goes wrong in people who can't make NO, we must break down each step in the pathway. The first step in the entero-salivary circulation of nitrate and production of nitric oxide is to make sure we get enough nitrate from our diet through consumption of green leafy vegetables. The next step involves the activation of nitrate into nitrite and nitric oxide by bacteria. Nitrate is inert in the human body, meaning that humans cannot utilize this molecule since we do not have the enzyme systems necessary to activate it. The process of converting nitrate to nitrite and nitric oxide is dependent upon select and specific bacteria that live in and on our body—at least a dozen or more types, according to research.

It has also been shown that people who do not have these bacteria in their mouth become nitric oxide deficient, and are thus at increased risk for developing cardiovascular disease. In fact, it has been shown that if you use a mouthwash that kills oral bacteria for seven days, your blood pressure will go up. This is profound. Who would have thought that mouthwash could affect your blood pressure? The observation that killing oral bacteria causes an increase in blood pressure reveals without a doubt that there are specific bacteria that are helpful and beneficial in generating nitric oxide. So, if you are taking an antiseptic mouthwash, my recommendation is that you stop. It is better to have bad breath than to have a heart attack. Statistics based on the U.S. Census data and Simmons National Consumer Survey (NHCS) show that 188.2 million Americans used mouthwash/dental rinse in 2011. This figure was projected to increase to 206.35 million in 2020.

This suggests that more than half of the U.S. population may not be getting a physiological response from dietary nitrate consumption, either from consuming green leafy vegetables or from drinking nitrate-enriched beetroot juice. To put this clearly, one can never get all the health benefits of eating a good diet rich in green leafy vegetables if these bacteria are lacking. From the previous chapter, we know that many of the health-promoting benefits of green leafy vegetables are due to their nitrate content. However, if we do not have the right bacteria to activate the nitrate into a usable form for nitric oxide generation, then we will never get all the health benefits of vegetables. We will still get the other nutrients and vitamins that vegetables provide—but without the nitric oxide benefit, we lose many of their heart-healthy properties.

The many health benefits of this newly discovered pathway are clear. Eating vegetables or consuming beetroot juice has been shown to lower blood pressure, improve exercise performance, improve blood vessel function and elasticity, improve cognition in aging patients with pre-Alzheimer's disease or vascular dementia, and basically combat all aspects of aging. Interestingly, all these effects are lost if the subjects do not swallow their own saliva or if nitrate is removed from the vegetables or beet juice. Remember when your mother told you as a child to eat your vegetables and do not spit? This was actually very good advice, since this will promote NO production. This is clear evidence of the importance of nitrate in our diet and having the right systems functional in our bodies to be able to utilize nitrate to generate nitric oxide.

To summarize, vegetables that contain dietary nitrate that may be converted to nitric oxide in the body. However, this requires a certain threshold of nitrate and the right oral nitrate-reducing bacteria to reduce nitrate to nitrite. Once nitrite is concentrated in the saliva and swallowed, it generates nitric oxide in the acid environment of the stomach. Therefore, vegetables can be a source of nitric oxide, but require all three phases to be efficient. Below are limitations and problems with just using vegetables to restore nitric oxide:

1. **All vegetables aren't created equal.** Depending on what type of vegetable and where the vegetables are grown and the soil conditions, they may or may not contain sufficient nitrate for nitric oxide production. Nitrate content of many vegetables has been measured and quantified, and some contain no nitrate at all. Since there is no standardization of nitrate in vegetables, just consuming any vegetable does not guarantee you will be getting nitrate.

2. **Lack of oral nitrate-reducing bacteria.** Based on our studies, we estimate that 30 to 40 percent of the population does not have the right oral nitrate-reducing bacteria. This is due primarily to use of antibiotics and antiseptic mouthwash. Also, people with poor oral hygiene do not appear to have the right bacteria—likely due to being out-competed for resources by disease-causing bacteria.

3. **Lack of stomach acid production.** Most people take an antacid medication that suppresses stomach acid production. There is also an age-related decline in stomach

acid production due to insufficient zinc and iodine in the diet or uptake in the stomach.

While there are limitations, we have shown that simply providing more nitrate through the diet is sufficient for changing the oral microbial communities and providing a more favorable environment for them to grow. Having the right nitrate-reducing bacteria will generate nitrite and nitric oxide. Most, if not all, pathogenic bacteria are sensitive to NO. Therefore, restoring the oral cavity with good nitrate-reducing bacteria will help eradicate the bad bacteria.

You should also make sure the vegetables you eat contain sufficient nitrate. Vegetables like kale, spinach, arugula, beets, cabbage, and many other green leafy vegetables typically have the highest nitrate content. Making sure you have sufficient stomach acid is another critical consideration. Taking a teaspoon of apple cider vinegar prior to meals will help acidify the stomach and lead to better digestion and more NO production from your diet. Apple cider vinegar is acetic acid that has a pH of around 2. You need a stomach pH of less than 3 in order to optimize NO production. If you are taking antacids, make every effort to stop and get off these medications. They were never designed to be used daily or for more than a couple of days at a time. As you will learn, anything that disrupts nitric oxide production is very damaging to your health. To summarize:

1. Eat more green leafy vegetables.

2. Stop using mouthwash and don't overuse antibiotics.

3. Make sure your stomach is making stomach acid.

These three simple lifestyle modifications will significantly improve your nitric oxide production.

- 4 -

Bacteria: Helping Us Do What We Cannot Do

Most people think of bacteria as infectious disease causing organisms. While there are some harmful bacteria that can make humans sick, most of the bacteria that live in and on our body are essential for our own health. In fact the number of bacteria that live in and on our body outnumber human cells by a factor of ten. Yes, there are over 10 times more bacteria cells than our own cells. These bacteria are what are referred to as symbiotic bacteria, meaning that they benefit and the human host benefits from their metabolic activity. In essence, they do essential biochemistry or perform reactions that humans cannot do thereby providing essential nutrients or molecules for normal human physiology. The human microbiome is composed of many different bacterial species, which outnumber our human cells ten to one and provide functions that are essential for our survival. Most of the research over the past couple decades has focused on the gut microbiome. The bacteria of the lower intestinal tract play an essential role in maintaining a healthy body. In fact, many people take a probiotic to help restore gut bacteria, to aid in digestion and even combat a number of diseases. These bacteria are necessary for nutrient acquisition and bile acid recycling, among other activities. Less studied are the oral bacteria. It has been known for many years and even decades that oral pathogens related to periodontal disease and gingivitis can also cause cardiovascular disease. As discussed in previous chapters, a human nitrogen cycle has been identified. This pathway, termed entero-salivary nitrate-nitrite-nitric oxide pathway, can positively affect nitric oxide production and represents a potential symbiotic relationship between oral bacteria and their human hosts—meaning that the bacteria are performing essential metabolic steps that we as humans cannot perform.

As a result, both the bacteria and the human hosts benefit. The oral commensal bacteria provide an important metabolic function in human physiology by contributing a source of nitric oxide. As we learned earlier, NO is one of the most important molecules produced in the human body. This bacterial process is analogous to the environmental nitrogen cycle whereby soil bacteria convert atmospheric nitrogen from fertilizers to usable forms for plant growth. Human nitrate reduction requires the presence of nitrate-reducing bacteria, as mammalian cells cannot effectively reduce this anion. The discovery of the NO pathway in the 1980s represented a critical advance in understanding cardiovascular disease, and today a number of human diseases are characterized by NO insufficiency. There is sufficient and convincing evidence in the literature that these bacterial communities provide the host a source of NO that may be able to overcome insufficient NO production from the blood vessels. The focus of this chapter is to discuss the new science of oral bacterial nitrate reduction, providing humans with a rescue pathway for conditions of NO insufficiency and diseases associated with NO insufficiency.

Nitrate that is concentrated in our saliva after we eat a meal with green leafy vegetables or beetroot juice has to be metabolized to nitrite, a reaction that human cells are unable to perform. Manipulation of the bacteria as a therapeutic target for disease management is on the near horizon. In fact, you have probably heard of fecal transplants, where doctors can take bacteria from the fecal matter of a healthy person and transplant it into the colon of a sick person with great success and change the bacteria profile from "bad" to "good". I predict this will be similar for oral bacteria, whereby people with good oral microbiome can donate a portion of their bacteria to be transplanted or inoculated into those people who may not have the right oral bacteria. The mouth cavity is an attractive target for probiotic and/or prebiotic therapy because of the ease of access.

Although a few nitrate-reducing bacteria in the oral cavity have been identified, we are just now beginning to identify which bacteria are necessary and sufficient for nitric oxide production. Everyone has a different microbiome, and specific bacteria are associated with good nitrate reduction. These bacteria are: Granulicatella adiacens, Haemophilus parainfluenzae, Actinomyces odontolyticus, Actinomyces viscosus, Actinomyces oris, Neisseria flavescens, Neisseria mucosa, Neisseria sicca, Neisseria subflava, Prevotella melaninogenica, Prevotella salivae, Veillonella dispar, Veillonella parvula, and Veillonella atypica. Additionally, Fusobacterium nucleatum and Brevibacillus brevis were designated as species of interest even though they are typically at much lower abundance.

So, how do you know if you have the right bacteria? This is a fundamentally important question to ensuring your own health and preventing many age-related diseases due to nitric oxide deficiency. Since nitrite accumulates in saliva from the reduction of nitrate in the oral cavity, determining salivary nitrite concentrations may offer simple means to determine the presence or absence of nitrate-reducing bacteria.

However, understanding that nitrite in our saliva comes from NO produced within the lining of our blood vessels and also from reduction of nitrate by oral bacteria. There are steps in this pathway that can become disrupted and lead to changes in salivary nitrite. Each step is described below:

1. Nitrate (from oxidation of NO or diet) uptake in the gut and transport to salivary glands. This is dependent upon how much nitrate you get from your diet and how much NO your body makes.

2. Nitrate secretion by salivary glands: The volumes of saliva produced vary depending on the type and intensity of stimulation.

3. Oral bacterial nitrate reduction: Humans lack a functional nitrate reductase, so salivary nitrate reduction is dependent upon oral commensal nitrate-reducing bacteria.

4. Oral pH: Healthy oral pH is between 6.5 and 7.5. The pKa of nitrite is 3.4, which means that any pH around or lower than 3.4 nitrite will become NO. Therefore, any condition that lowers the pH in the oral cavity may destabilize nitrite and affect the use of salivary nitrite as a measure of nitrate reduction. We need an acidic environment in the stomach but not in the mouth.

There are now salivary test strips that measure the amount of nitrite in your saliva. Salivary nitrite is a biomarker for total body nitric oxide bioavailability. If your saliva is low in nitrite, then your body is low in nitric oxide. It could be that your blood vessels aren't making enough NO, or it could be that you don't have the right bacteria to metabolize nitrate to nitrite. Regardless of the issue, if you are low in salivary nitrite, then your body is low in NO. So, grab a test strip and apply your saliva to the test pad. Within a couple of seconds, the test strip will turn a shade of pink. The darker the pink/red color, the more NO you have. The lighter shade of pink is representative of low NO. If you test low, then go eat a salad—preferably a high nitrate salad with spinach, kale, etc. Approximately 90 to 120 minutes later, retest using the salivary test strip. If you improve the color on the test strip, then you have the right bacteria to convert the nitrate in the salad into nitrite and nitric oxide in your body. This is a good thing. If you do not improve the color on the test strip, then you do not have the right bacteria to convert the nitrate in your diet into nitric oxide.

If the latter is the case, what do you need to do? First, if you are taking a mouthwash, you should stop. Second, you should consume more nitrate-containing foods. The nitrate-reducing bacteria require nitrate in order to respire and colonize in the oral cavity. If you do not eat enough nitrate-rich vegetables, then you are not providing enough fuel for these bacteria to survive.

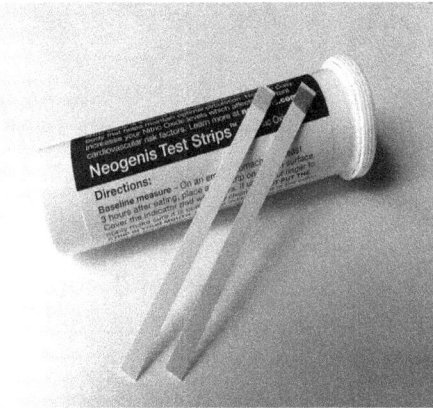

As a result of this human nitrogen cycle and enterosalivary circulation of nitrate (both from diet and endogenous NO production), and subsequent reduction to nitrite in the mouth, sampling salivary nitrite can be used as an accurate representation of the presence or absence of nitrate-reducing bacteria. Saliva offers a number of advantages as a biological compartment for diagnostics. There is sufficient evidence to show that increased circulating levels of plasma nitrite correlate with changes in blood pressure. Furthermore, blood and salivary levels of nitrite increase after a nitrate load, and killing the oral bacteria with a mouthwash or antibiotic causes a decrease in salivary nitrite and an increase in blood pressure. To the contrary, as NO availability is decreased, both plasma and salivary levels of nitrite decline. So, whether there is sufficient NO produced by the blood vessels (pathway 1, or the L-arginine pathway) to form nitrite and nitrate in the circulation—which is then concentrated in our salivary glands—or there is sufficient nitrate ingested in the diet (pathway 2, nitrate-nitrite-nitric oxide pathway), this will be reflected as nitrite in the saliva. Understanding the basis and rationale for sampling salivary nitrite as well as recognizing the limitations, physicians and patients can gain new information from this non-invasive diagnostic, including accurate assessment of total body NO availability, cardiovascular risk, and NO homeostasis. More research is needed in order to determine if this approach may have clinical utility. Salivary nitrite measurements may offer an indirect measure of the ability of humans to reduce nitrate.

The realization that bacteria in our mouth can affect our systemic health has been known for a while, but the realization that it is nitric oxide that may be responsible for this effect is groundbreaking. The potential to exploit the symbiotic nitrate-nitrite-NO pathway to NO production is profound, particularly because adequate and sustained control of blood pressure is achieved in only about 50 percent of treated hypertensive patients—including all classes of anti-hypertensives medication. Since NO is known to affect many other biological processes, this knowledge also has the potential to affect all chronic diseases. As cardiovascular disease remains the top killer in the U.S., accounting for more deaths each year than cancer, designing new diagnostics, treatments, and preventives for diseased and at-risk individuals is essential. This poses the question - Do people that have high blood pressure, simply have an oral microbiome problem? With over 50% of the people taking anti-hypertensive medications getting no response from these medications, this new concept may explain why. It's time to focus on the problem.

Additionally, because NO is an important signaling molecule in all body systems, exploiting the oral microbiome to contribute to NO production and maintain NO homeostasis has the potential to affect human health beyond the cardiovascular system.

Being able to repopulate essential nitrate-reducing bacteria in the oral cavity is of immense interest, since this may be an effective means to restore NO availability in the human body. Recent research in rats found that simply feeding nitrate in the diet could lead to a significant increase in nitrate-reducing Haemophilus parainfluenzae. Additionally, Granulicatella and Aggregatibacter, which have both been associated with poor oral health in humans, decreased with additional nitrate in the diet. These results suggest that high nitrate diets may induce changes in oral microbiome communities to more efficiently reduce nitrate to nitrite and NO, which could be beneficial both for reducing blood pressure and inhibiting bacterial species associated with poor oral health. Since nitrite and NO are toxic to many pathogenic bacteria, simply adding more nitrate in the form of green leafy vegetables may allow for restoring the balance of good vs bad bacteria. This suggests that dietary nitrate and nitrite may act as a prebiotic for the oral microbiome.

For the past thirty years, scientists have focused on NO production/regulation at the level of nitric oxide synthase (NOS), pathway 1 described earlier from L-arginine. However, this pathway becomes dysfunctional with age and disease and produces less and less NO the older and sicker we get. The notion that this can be overcome by targeting oral bacteria is profound and revolutionary. Therapeutically, then, perhaps an effective strategy to promote NO production and overcome conditions of NO insufficiency may not be targeted at pathway 1 in the blood vessels, but rather on targeting specific oral nitrate-reducing bacterial communities. Understanding and harnessing this redundant compensatory pathway may prove to be a viable and cost-effective strategy. Furthermore, new research reveals that this may in fact be the biochemical and physiological link between oral health and cardiovascular disease through maintenance of NO production. Because NO signaling affects all organ systems and almost all disease processes described to date, this novel approach to NO regulation has the potential to affect the study and treatment of many diseases across all organ systems.

What is clear from this most recent research is that disruption of nitrite and NO production in the oral cavity may contribute to the oral-systemic link between oral hygiene and cardiovascular risk and disease. The identification of new biomarkers for NO insufficiency and the exploitation of the oral microbiota to increase cardiovascular health will be enabled by further characterization of the enzymatic activities of native oral bacterial communities from larger groups of people and specific patient populations. These groups should consist not only of a specific U.S. population, but also of others (European, Asian). It is likely that the oral microbiomes of different ethnic groups, even those within different regions of the U.S., vary widely. It will be important to determine whether different nitrate-reducing communities are more prevalent in geographically dispersed healthy populations; likewise, it will also be important to determine whether different nitrate-reducing communities are lacking in specific patient populations from around the world.

If certain patient populations lack specific nitrate-reducing bacteria, personalized treatments to enrich for nitrate reducers may be warranted. Is it tempting to wonder whether the use of mouthwash may be discouraged as part of such treatments. Indeed, studies have shown that using mouthwash raises blood pressure in humans. Additionally, while antibiotics are sometimes used to target specific bacterial species, it is possible that potential deleterious effects of antibiotic usage on nitrate-reducing communities may preclude the use of antibiotics in specific patient populations.

Clearly, the potential for the entero-salivary nitrate-nitrite-NO pathway (pathway 2) to serve as a NO bioavailability maintenance system by harnessing the nitrate reductase activity of specific commensal bacteria calls may be profound and truly transformative. Future studies are likely to unveil new paradigms on the regulation and production of endogenous NO that are likely to be new targets for specialized, multi-faceted, and potentially personalized therapeutic interventions. These studies will have the potential to: 1) redefine the meaning of "healthy oral microbiome" to include microbes associated with NO production, 2) provide a new target for NO-based therapies and open a new direction in cardiovascular research, and 3) allow development of new diagnostics targeted at specific oral microbial communities or select bacteria, the absence of which may reflect a state of NO insufficiency and change the treatment strategies for NO restoration in a number of different diseases. This is the focus of my current research program. With the loss of NO signaling and homeostasis being one of the earliest events in the onset and progression of cardiovascular disease, targeting microbial communities early in the process may lead to better preventative interventions in cardiovascular medicine. This may also affect the way oral health professionals recommend hygienic practices.

- 5 -

Focus on Nitrogen-Based Nutrients

The atmosphere and environment on Earth is made up of 78 percent nitrogen (N2). Nitrogen is a vital macronutrient for plants, necessary for basic cellular function and production of many basic cellular components, such as DNA, RNA, and proteins. It is also an essential nutrient for plant growth, development, and reproduction. Plants need nitrogen in a form that is usable by the plant for growth, since they are unable to utilize elemental nitrogen or N2. Nitrogen itself is not directly available to plants, but some can be converted to available forms by microorganisms found in the soil or from decaying matter. Despite nitrogen being one of the most abundant elements on Earth, nitrogen deficiency is probably the most common nutritional problem affecting plants worldwide, and perhaps nitrogen in the form of nitrate or nitrite may be the most common nutritional problem affecting humans worldwide. This is because both plants and humans must have the right form of nitrogen.

Soil nitrogen exists in three general forms: organic nitrogen compounds, ammonium (NH_4^+) ions, and nitrate (NO_3^-) ions. At any given time, 95 to 99 percent of the potentially available nitrogen in the soil is in organic forms, meaning decaying plant and animal residues. Nitrogen in the form of nitrate or ammonia is taken up by plants through roots from inorganic or organic sources, such as amino acids. In agricultural settings, nitrogen may be a limiting factor for plant growth and yield. That is why nitrogen-based fertilizers are added to crops and fields. A plant deficient in this nitrogen will shunt resources away from its shoot in order to expand its root system and acquire more nitrogen. Most plants take nitrogen from the soil continuously throughout their lives, and nitrogen demand usually increases as plant size increases.

A plant supplied with adequate nitrogen and has the capabilities to fix and assimilate nitrogen into ammonia. Nitrate causes plants to grow rapidly and produces large amounts of succulent, green foliage and vegetables. Adequate nitrogen allows an annual crop, such as corn, to grow to full maturity on time. A nitrogen-deficient plant is generally small and develops slowly because it lacks the nitrogen necessary to manufacture adequate structural and genetic materials. It is usually pale green or yellowish because it lacks adequate chlorophyll. Older leaves often become necrotic and die as the plant moves nitrogen from less important older tissues to more important younger ones. In nature, wildfires, although devastating at times, do provide nature's way of putting nitrogen back into the soil. Farmers often burn crops and hay fields to naturally replenish nitrogen making for beautiful lush, green grass & crops. Again, nature has a tendency to take care of itself.

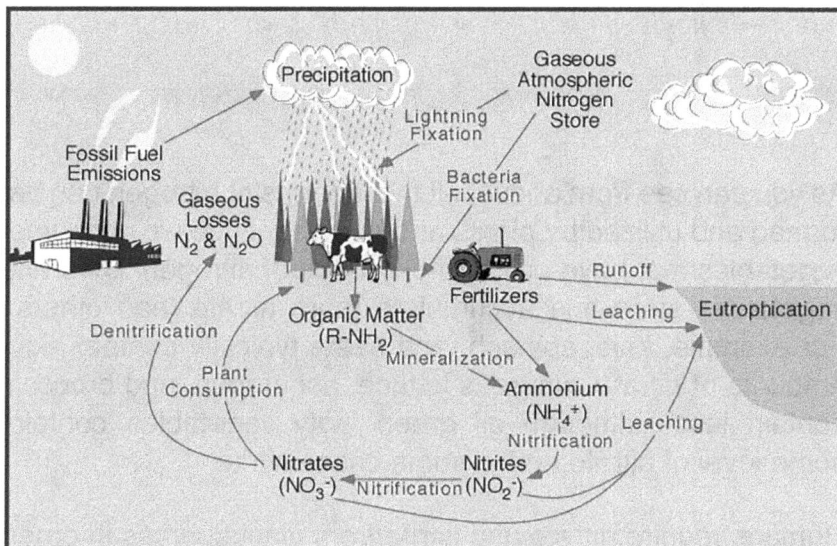

Early experiments in herbivores in the 1830s proposed that the relative nutritional values of plant foods could be assessed from their contents of nitrogen. The scientists concluded that foods that do not contain some form of nitrogen cannot continue to support life. Most plants have bacteria or fungi in the root systems that can fix nitrogen into usable forms for energy. For plants that do not have a symbiont partner to provide them with fixed nitrogen, nitrate, found in soil, is the preferred source of fixed nitrogen. Therefore, any plant or vegetable grown in soil accumulates primarily nitrate, but also to a lesser extent nitrite. So, when we eat vegetables, we consume nitrate, an essential nutrient. Although plants can use nitrate as a form of energy, humans cannot make use of nitrate. It must first be metabolized by bacteria that live in and on the human body. This was discussed in the previous chapter.

Nitrogen fixation is a reversible process that can be harnessed based on specific needs of plants and also humans.

$$NO_3- \rightarrow NO_2- \rightarrow NO \rightarrow N_2O \rightarrow N_2 \rightarrow NH_3$$

| Nitrate | Nitrite | Nitric Oxide | Nitrous Oxide | Nitrogen | Ammonia |

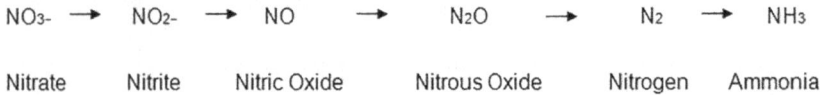

As you can see from above, all these forms of nitrogen can be formed and utilized by plants and humans, once we consume vegetables that have one or more forms of nitrogen. Different vegetables store and accumulate more nitrate than others. For example, kale, spinach, and beets typically contain high amounts of nitrate, whereas lettuce, asparagus, and broccoli contain less—although all green leafy vegetables contain some level of nitrate and in some cases nitrite.

Humans require nitrate and nitrite from plant sources in order to make nitric oxide. Just as in plants, humans require sources of nitrogen to make amino acids. These form proteins, to make DNA and to maintain normal metabolism. Therefore, nitrogen-based nutrients in the form of nitrate and nitrite are essential for human health and disease prevention.

- 6 -

Why Vegetables are Good for You

We have been told since we were kids to "Eat your vegetables." Our moms and grandmas insisted we eat vegetables, and most kids hate vegetables. However, your mom was right. We should eat our vegetables, and we should eat them at every meal. So, we have established that vegetables are good for you. But perhaps we have missed the most important reason vegetables are good for you. It is because they provide the human body with nitrate and nitrite, which we discussed in the previous chapter. There are scientific truths and facts that cannot be denied or ignored. Any diet that is not based on sound scientific evidence or rationale will always come and go and be a "fad". Diets and foods are the most important determinant of your health. Nothing affects your health more than what you eat. Our body is designed to get all the nutrients and material it needs from our diet. Diets that eliminate certain food groups that provide essential nutrients will never be sustaining. To the contrary, diets that provide a balance of nutrients to replete what the human body is missing will be the most nutritious and helpful for human health. There are a number of diets that have proven to be healthy, and their common denominator is that they provide sufficient nitrite and nitrate for optimal wellness. These include the Mediterranean diet, South Beach Diet, Dietary Approaches to Stop Hypertension (DASH), and Paleo. All of these diets recommend consumption of several servings of vegetables, particularly green leafy vegetables, in their meal plans. So what is it about these diets that allows them to survive the test of time and remain at the top of the list of the best diets out there?

The DASH diet is a clinically researched diet rich in fruits, vegetables (especially green, leafy ones), low-fat dairy foods, and with reduced saturated and total fat that can substantially lower blood pressure. This diet is commonly used by those interested in supporting healthy blood pressure levels through the food they eat. The Mediterranean diet recommends emulating how people in the Mediterranean region have traditionally eaten, with a focus on foods like olive oil, fish and vegetables. U.S. News and World Report called the diet a "well-balanced eating plan" and pointed to research that suggests the diet helps prevent some major chronic diseases and increases longevity. The heart-healthy nature of all these diets are due to the fact that they provide more dietary nitrite and nitrate than the standard Western diet. We have analyzed the foods from all these diet plans and found that one can easily meet and exceed the accepted daily intake of nitrite and nitrate.

Epidemiology is the branch of medicine that deals with the incidence, distribution, and possible control of diseases and other factors relating to health. Nutritional epidemiology is an area of epidemiology that involves research to examine the role of nutrition in the etiology of disease, monitor the nutritional status of populations, and develop and evaluate interventions to achieve and maintain healthy eating patterns among populations. Most, if not all, epidemiological studies investigating green leafy vegetables show that these foods protect from cancer, cardiovascular disease, Alzheimer's disease, and many other chronic diseases. For years, scientists believed this association was due to the rich source of antioxidants and vitamins vegetables provide. However, when clinical studies are conducted investigating the individual vitamins and antioxidants found in these vegetables, they fail to reproduce the protective effects of the vegetables themselves. Therefore, there must be an "unknown nutrient" in these vegetables that is responsible for the protective effects.

A meta-analysis is a statistical technique for combining the findings from independent studies. Meta-analysis of antioxidant supplements affecting a number of diseases reveal there is no benefit in fighting most diseases. Meta-analysis is most often used to assess the clinical effectiveness of healthcare interventions. It does this by combining data from two or more randomized control trials. The current evidence does not support the use of antioxidant supplements in the general population or in patients with various diseases. So, what is it about vegetables that clearly show protection from cardiovascular disease, cancer, Alzheimer's, and most chronic diseases?

Is nitrate the answer?

That's the question an international team of scientists from the world-famous Karolinska Institute in Sweden and from Boston University School of Medicine asked themselves while wondering why vegetables protect the heart from disease. Their scientific paper in the medical journal Nitric Oxide—"Cardioprotective effects of vegetables: Is nitrate the answer?"—offers this perspective:

1. Eating a diet rich in vegetables lowers blood pressure almost as much as treatment with a standard pressure-lowering drug.

2. The high content of nitrate in certain vegetables, and its conversion to nitrite and NO, is the real reason why vegetables are cardioprotective.

3. In fact, this pathway of NO generation works better than the L-arginine pathway, which "malfunctions" in people with heart disease.

4. Vegetarians (who have low rates of heart disease) consume about 10 times more nitrate than nonvegetarians, as do people who eat a Mediterranean-style diet, also shown to protect against heart disease.

5. The task for scientists is to find the optimal level of nitrate and nitrite intake for cardioprotection.

Their conclusions:

1. "The protective effect of certain vegetables on the cardiovascular system is related to their high content of nitrate."

2. "The mechanism involves reduction of dietary nitrate to nitrite [and] nitric oxide."

3. "A continuous intake of nitrate-containing food such as green leafy vegetables may ensure that tissue levels of NO . . . are maintained."

4. "If proven true, these considerations could have a profound impact on our view of the role of diet . . . in the . . . prevention of cardiovascular disease."

They took the words right out of our mouths!

The evidence now supports the fact that nitrate and nitrite may be the active nutrients in vegetables that make them so healthy. Unlike vitamins and antioxidants like vitamins C, E, and A, which have failed to show positive effects in clinical trials, studies over the past fifteen years investigating nitrite and/or nitrate have undeniably demonstrated that these nutrients can in fact protect from heart disease, lower blood pressure, improve athletic performance, improve Alzheimer's, and more. Several studies reveal that a single serving of leafy green vegetables each day may help keep dementia away. In one study, researchers evaluated the eating habits and mental ability of more than 950 older adults for an average of five years. They found that those who consumed one or two servings of foods such as spinach, kale, mustard greens, and/or collards daily experienced slower mental deterioration than those who ate no leafy greens at all. The researchers suggested that it may be due to the vitamin K provided specifically by these leafy greens. However, I do not think it is a coincidence that these are the foods most enriched in nitrate.

Diets rich in fruits and vegetables are consistently associated with a decreased risk of cancer. The U.S. federal government has embraced this tenet as evidenced in the Healthy People 2000 and Healthy People 2010 campaigns, which advocated the consumption of five or more servings of fruits and vegetables daily. In addition, the National Cancer Institute (NCI), in conjunction with the Produce for Better Health Foundation, implemented the National 5 A Day for Better Health Program in 1991 to encourage Americans to eat five or more servings of fruits and vegetables every day in the context of a healthy diet. These initiatives have led to Americans consuming more fruits and vegetables, but they are not regularly consuming the particular fruits and vegetables that are likely to impart robust health effects. Specifically, they are not eating enough dark green leafy vegetables, those with high amounts of nitrate and nitrite.

What is clear from nutritional epidemiology is that people who eat lots of green leafy vegetables are typically healthier than those who do not eat green leafy vegetables. What then is the active nutrient or compound that could account for the impressive health benefits of vegetables? The answer is clearly and undeniably nitrate. The previous chapters have revealed how nitrate is taken up and then metabolized into nitrite and nitric oxide by oral nitrate-reducing bacteria and stomach acid production. So, to this point, we know that nitric oxide is absolutely essential for optimal health and disease prevention. We know nitrogen in the form of nitrate in our foods is good, if we have the right oral bacteria to metabolize nitrate into nitrite and nitric oxide. So, what do the published clinical studies tell us on what we can expect from functional nitric oxide nutrition? The next chapter will reveal just that.

- 7 -

Undisputed Health Benefits

Sufficient nitric oxide production is crucial for the maintenance of every organ system in the human body, and the body cannot function optimally without it. In fact, every single chronic disease involves loss of nitric oxide production. Whether it is glaucoma, macular degeneration, vascular dementia, Alzheimer's disease, heart disease, kidney disease, liver disease, diabetes, stroke, or even cancer, all of these conditions are characterized by a loss of sufficient blood flow to the respective organs or tissues that does not allow them to function properly. As a result, they fail. This then creates a very simple model for treating, curing, and preventing most if not all chronic diseases. Restore blood supply to the organs by fixing the nitric oxide production pathways, so blood vessels then have a way to dilate and bring new oxygen and nutrients to these starved tissues. The million-dollar question, then, is how do we do this?

When our body makes nitric oxide, nitrite is the main stable product of NO in plasma. The amount of nitrite in the blood reflects acute and chronic changes in NO production. Although it is very difficult to measure NO directly in the blood, increases in nitrite in the blood after an increase in NO production is an effective way to measure one's ability to produce NO from the L-arginine pathway. Therefore, people who are deficient in NO are deficient in nitrite. It has been shown that exercise increases nitrite in healthy people. To the contrary, older unhealthy individuals—who are unable to produce NO when they exercise—fail to increase nitrite and also fail an exercise stress test. This is diagnostic for heart disease. Under fasting conditions, the ability to increase plasma nitrite in response to exercise actually predicts how well one can perform . Age-dependent alterations of the structure and function of blood vessels predispose older individuals to increased risk of cardiovascular disease.

Similarly, if your body can't make NO when you begin to exercise, this is a critical determinant of your risk for heart disease. This usually becomes evident in people ages 60 and over when they go for a routine exercise stress test. Similarly, when you engage in sexual activity, you need an increase in blood flow to the sex organs to get and maintain an erection. This is true for both men and women. So, if your body cannot make NO before or during sexual activity (which is physical exercise), then you develop sexual dysfunction or erectile dysfunction. Again, this is diagnostic for more serious vascular concerns that indicate your body does not make sufficient NO. This can occur much earlier, sometimes in late 30s and early 40s. With over 50 percent of men over the age of 40 showing symptoms of some degree of erectile dysfunction, this is the first sign of insufficient NO production and allows time for nutritional intervention. Functional nitric oxide nutrition can be a very effective strategy to overcome these age-related and other disruptions in vascular NO production.

This raises the question as to whether providing more nitrite and nitrate in the diet can restore NO-based signaling and functions. The answer to this question has transformed science and medicine over the past twenty years. These discoveries have shed new light on how the human body makes NO, and more importantly provided safe and effective dietary strategies (functional nitric oxide nutrition) to restore NO insufficiency. Dietary nitrite and/or nitrate can provide a reservoir of NO activity and the ability to produce NO from the blood vessels.

Hopefully by now you can appreciate the importance of NO and the serious health consequences that occur when your body cannot make sufficient NO. The concept of functional nitric oxide nutrition can provide the human body with a source of NO that it otherwise cannot produce, and also fix the underlying problems of why people cannot make sufficient NO. Drug therapy does not do this. Only functional nutrition can do this. Simply providing more nitrite and nitrate in the diet, and fixing the broken systems that allow for the metabolism of nitrate to nitrite and nitrite to NO, has shown remarkable results in human clinical trials. Over the past ten years, there have been many published studies showing health benefits in humans supplementing dietary nitrite and nitrate, including blood pressure regulation and sports performance. For the majority of studies in humans, investigators used beetroot juice—standardized to a known amount of nitrate. The findings show that increasing plasma nitrite levels can increase NO production and improve oxygen efficiency and athletic performance.

In studies in older adults, nitrate supplementation with beetroot juice reduced blood pressure and positively influenced exercise capacity. Even in patients with peripheral artery disease, nitrate supplementation improved exercise performance, whereas L-arginine was ineffective in these patients. This demonstrates that the nitrate-nitrite-nitric oxide pathway can rescue and overcome disruptions in the L-arginine pathway. Dietary nitrate can also lower blood pressure. Drinking a bottle of beetroot juice containing nitrate lowers blood pressure six hours later in healthy adults.

Antiseptic mouthwash eradicates the benefits of nitrate

When relying on nitrate alone from dietary sources, there are a number of steps in the process that can become disrupted and will not allow the nitric oxide mediated benefits from nitrate. All the health benefits of nitrate are completely abolished if people taking nitrate are not allowed to swallow or if they use an antiseptic mouthwash to kill oral bacteria. Studies have shown that use of antiseptic mouthwash for seven days caused a decrease in salivary and plasma nitrite, with an increase in systolic and diastolic blood pressure, demonstrating the removal of these bacteria with an antibacterial mouthwash will very likely block the NO-dependent biological effects of dietary nitrate.

Over 180 million Americans use mouthwash on a daily basis, and in 2015 alone, approximately 269 million antibiotic prescriptions were dispensed from outpatient pharmacies in the United States—enough for five out of every six people to receive one antibiotic prescription each year. Interestingly, at least 30 percent of these antibiotic prescriptions were unnecessary. Use of both antiseptic mouthwash and antibiotics disrupts the oral microbiome and leads to a complete lack of nitrate reduction, or at least a decreased efficiency of nitrate reduction and conversion to nitrite.

Also, given the diversity and variability of the oral microbiome between certain individuals and cultures, it is uncertain how many people have the correct nitrate-reducing bacteria. With prevalence of antibiotic and antiseptic mouthwash use in the U.S. along with periodontal disease and poor oral hygiene, it would not be surprising if over half of the population is unable to reduce dietary nitrate. This means that although they may be consuming what is considered a healthy diet even with sufficient nitrate, they are unable to get a nitric oxide benefit due to lack of nitrate reduction and conversion to nitrite by bacteria. This should be a new consideration in patient assessment.

Stomach acid is required for optimal NO production

Even if you have the right oral nitrate-reducing bacteria, this does not always mean you will get a benefit from the nitrate consumed in your diet. Stomach acid is required for optimal effects of salivary nitrite. Nitrite concentration in the saliva from reduction of dietary nitrate when swallowed becomes protonated (nitrite pKa ~ 3.4) to form nitrous acid and nitric oxide. Proton pump inhibitors (PPIs), a type of antacid used by people with acid reflux, shuts down NO production by inhibiting stomach acid production and increasing gastric pH—which will prevent formation of nitrous acid from inorganic nitrite, and, in turn, NO release. Indeed, studies have shown that taking antacids will block the blood pressure lowering effects of orally administered sodium nitrite. Furthermore, PPIs blunt the favorable effects of antioxidants on nitrite-to-NO conversion in the stomach. PPIs also specifically lead to the accumulation of asymmetric dimethyl L-arginine (ADMA).

ADMA is generated during metabolism of cellular proteins consumed through the diet. ADMA is broken down by the enzyme dimethylarginine dimethylaminohydrolase, found in many cells. The inhibition of the DDAH enzyme is the major contributor to increases in ADMA in animal models and patients with cardiovascular risk factors. Evidence now demonstrates that PPI drugs directly inhibit DDAH activity. In addition to inhibiting DDAH, PPIs affect the amount of the enzyme that normally produces NO that is present in cells. So, they actually decrease the amount of NO the body can produce. Altogether, these findings provide direct proof that antacid drugs decrease nitric oxide production.

Studies published several years ago reveal that people who have taken antacid drugs for three to five years had about 30 percent more heart attacks and strokes. This is a huge effect. Imagine all the people who could benefit from this information. There are approximately 64.6 million prescriptions written for gastroesophageal reflux disease (GERD) medications in the

United States on an annual basis, accounting for over $11 billion in total healthcare expenditures in the U.S.—and this does not even include the over the counter (OTC) market. Any therapy that increases stomach pH will interrupt NO generation from salivary nitrite. Clear evidence is emerging that PPIs have adverse cardiovascular effects. These effects may be mediated primarily or at least in part through a disruption in NO production/signaling. They should be considered when PPIs are prescribed, especially in patients at increased cardiovascular risk.

It is important at this point to explain the difference in nitrate and nitrite. Nitrate is inert in humans, meaning that humans cannot metabolize this molecule and if it is not first metabolized by bacteria, then the body will just excrete nitrate through the sweat, urine, and feces. Although humans rely solely on bacteria to reduce nitrate to nitrite, we do have systems in place to generate nitric oxide from nitrite. Studies conducted by my research group in collaboration with Dr. David Lefer were the first to show that supplementing nitrite and/or nitrate in the diet protects the heart from injury from a heart attack. Not only can it protect the heart from injury, but research has shown it can protect the liver, the kidney, the brain, and most organs. We were also the first to show that nitrite in the diet can suppress inflammation, one of the hallmarks of all chronic diseases.

Nitrite prevents the oxidation of lipids, which is critically important in the development of heart disease. Nitrite in saliva that is then swallowed is important in controlling foodborne infection and in maintaining a healthy stomach lining. Long-term dietary nitrite causes formation of new blood vessels, which is important for people with peripheral artery disease and conditions of low blood flow such as diabetes. Nitrite in the form of an orally disintegrating tablet—with natural product chemistry to reduce nitrite to NO—has been shown to modify most if not all cardiovascular risk factors in people over the age of 40, reduce blood pressure, and reduce markers of inflammation. Since a substantial portion of steady state nitrite concentrations in blood and tissue are derived from dietary sources, supplementing nitrite in the diet can provide a first line of defense for conditions associated with NO insufficiency.

- 8 -

But I Thought Nitrite and Nitrate Were Toxic

Sometimes when we hear information repeated often enough, we start to believe it—whether we intend to or not. Remember being cautioned not to sit too close to the television or it would ruin your sight? How about the warning not to swallow gum because it would stay in your body for three years? While intuitively we know that we need to let these notions go, there's something about these repeated warnings that causes doubt to linger.

As a physiologist, I interact with a lot of people about how we can maintain healthy bodies. Increasingly, I hear misguided claims about food—like the idea that nitrite needs to be avoided or that the best way to avoid it is to stop eating cured meats like hot dogs and bacon. In some respects, it's understandable. People have heard cautions about nitrite for decades, especially claims that nitrite could cause cancer. But what people don't understand is its critical role not only in preventing foodborne illnesses, but most recently its recognized health benefits due to its ability to form nitric oxide or NO. Up until the 1970s, it was thought that nitrite and nitrate were synthetic unnatural molecules, but we soon realized that nitrite is actually produced in the bodies of mammals through normal metabolic processes. This realization is what ultimately led to the discovery of nitric oxide. Three American scientists were awarded the 1998 Nobel Prize for the discovery of nitric oxide. Now we know and appreciate the essential nature of both nitric oxide and nitrite in human health and disease.

The claim that nitrite and nitrate are toxic and should be avoided is particularly frustrating to me, because I know through my work and the work of others that much of what is reported in the previous chapters is true—that not only are nitrite and nitrate safe, but absolutely essential for life. Published studies reveal that these can protect from injury from heart attack and stroke, prevent inflammation from a poor diet, and even lower blood pressure, the primary risk factor for the development of cardiovascular disease. In fact, there are currently twenty-six clinical trials completed or ongoing using nitrite as a therapy for conditions like heart failure, organ transplantation, cystic fibrosis, and even leg ulcers just to name a few. Obviously, the scientific and medical community understand the importance of nitrite for human health—but the media sometimes mislead us or sensationalize certain stories.

Still, claims that "no nitrite is added" appear increasingly on foods these days, as if to suggest there is something to fear. There's just one catch: cured meats must contain a form of nitrite to be cured, or ham and salami would just be, well . . . pork. Most often, nitrite takes the form of celery powder or celery juice. Sometimes its sea salt or even beet juice, which are all rich sources of nitrate and nitrite. That's right—nitrite is found naturally in sea salt and most vegetables.

Now, here's the real shocker for most people: Less than five percent of the nitrite we consume comes from cured meats.

Approximately half of our daily nitrite intake comes from fruits, vegetables, and human saliva. The other half of our body's nitrite exposure comes from the production of nitric oxide, one of the most important molecules our body makes. Nitric oxide is then metabolized to nitrite. So, our body makes nitrite as part of its normal, healthy nitrogen cycle.

Studies have now shown that the health benefits of a Vegetarian diet, the Mediterranean diet, the Japanese diet, and the DASH (Dietary Approaches to Stop Hypertension) diet are due to the nitrite and nitrate found naturally in the foods consumed through these dietary patterns. Nitrite is also found naturally in breast milk, nature's most perfect food. Everything we know about nutrition and dietary patterns, from nursing infants to adults, demonstrates that nitrite and nitrate are absolutely essential for health and wellness. People who get more nitrite and nitrate from their diet have less disease. People who do not get sufficient nitrite and nitrate from their diet, or are unable to make nitric oxide, are more susceptible to disease.

Where did the nitrite controversy originate? A single study in the late 1970s claimed to have found increased tumors in lab rodents who were given nitrite along with a chemical that could react with nitrite (that chemical, by the way, is never found naturally in our food supply). The study's findings were never confirmed in follow-up research. However, given the controversy, the U.S. government's National Toxicology Program completed a study in 2000 in which rats and mice were fed nitrate and nitrite in their drinking water. Recipe for cancer? Not at all. The results published in 2001 concluded that there was no evidence of carcinogenicity (or cancer-causing activity) by nitrite at any dose. In fact, there was actually a decrease in the incidences of mononuclear cell leukemia in male and female rats. The researchers also concluded there was no issue at all with nitrate or nitrite in causing cancer.

A panel that reviewed the NTP study's findings voted and concluded that based on the data, nitrite is not a carcinogen at the levels used. The levels used in the study were far greater than what could ever be consumed in the diet, but still showed no evidence of cancer. That's why nitrite is NOT on the list of carcinogens maintained by the U.S. Certainly, there have been studies that report nitrite-containing foods like bacon and salami pose a health risk, but these are the same type of studies that ask people to recall what they ate and then analyze the data. They don't occur in laboratories where intake can be monitored and controlled. Remember, also, that people consume diets—not single foods—and memories about what was eaten are notoriously inaccurate.

The emergence and prevalence of "dietary nitrate" in products within the marketplace has created a lot of confusion. The confusion arises because for the past fifty years, we have been told to avoid nitrate-containing products such as cured and processed meats. So now, we are supposed to supplement our diet with nitrate? This transformation is called scientific progress. We know more now than we did fifty years ago. The truth is that over 80 percent of our dietary nitrate comes from green leafy and root vegetables. Only about 5 percent comes from cured and processed meats, and the other 15 percent comes from swallowing our own saliva. In fact, the reason vegetables are good for us is partly due to their dietary nitrate content and its metabolism to nitric oxide.

However, because there are biologically plausible mechanisms whereby nitrate or nitrite can cause nitrosamines, there are very effective strategies and mechanisms to prevent nitrosamine formation from nitrate or nitrite. The most effective is to have sufficient vitamin C present with any nitrite- or nitrate-containing food or nutritional product. Nature has included that level of protection in many vegetables. Most nitrate-rich vegetables are also enriched in vitamin C. Nitrate-based products without a specific amount of vitamin C may not confer the level of protection needed to prevent the formation of any and all nitrosamines. Perhaps the most convincing argument on the safety of nitrite and nitrate is the fact that both are enriched in human breast milk, nature's most perfect food. Nursing infants get a rich source of nitrite and nitrate, and that's one of the reasons that breastfed babies are typically healthier than formula-fed infants.

However, despite all the safety data, there are two safety concerns surrounding nitrite and nitrate. Acute toxicity is defined by methemoglobinemia; this is sometimes referred to as "Blue Baby Syndrome," or cyanosis. This occurs when nitrite causes oxidation of hemoglobin where it can no longer carry oxygen. As a result, blueness around the lips can occur due to lack of oxygenation. The fatal dose of nitrite is in the range of 22 to 23 mg/kg body weight, which would translate into about 1750 mg for a 180-pound adult. This dose is approximately 150 times higher than doses that have been used therapeutically in humans.

The other concern with nitrite and nitrate is the potential to form low molecular weight N-nitrosamines, some of which are carcinogenic. In the 1970s, there became a major public health concern regarding nitrite exposure, either through diet or industrial exposure, and formation of N-nitrosamines. The first report in the 1950s on the cancer-causing effects of N-nitrosodimethylamine (NDMA), and the suggestion that low molecular weight N-nitrosamines can be formed following nitrosation of various amines ignited an enormous interest in N-nitrosamines and their association with cancer. There are biologically plausible mechanisms that nitrite could form nitrosamines if you created a contrived environment. NDMA was detected in nitrite preserved fish. It was later demonstrated that nitrosamines could form in the acidic conditions of the human stomach. Since the early 1980s, there have been numerous reports on the association of N-nitrosamines and human cancers. More recent epidemiological evidence, as well as review of a biologically plausible mechanism, has refuted previous evidence of a causal relationship between nitrite and nitrate exposure and cancer formation. Despite this more recent evidence, there continues to be epidemiological studies demonstrating an association between dietary nitrite, nitrate intake, and certain forms of cancer.

As a physiologist, I'm trained to look at the big picture, and here's what I see. The NTP—the gold standard for assessing safety—found that nitrite did not cause cancer in a controlled study that was evaluated by a panel of experts. My research and many others', including researchers at the National Institutes of Health, have found nitrite to be an effective treatment for a number of health conditions without adverse effects. Our body makes nitrite. And vegetables like spinach, celery, cabbage, radishes, broccoli, rhubarb, and melons—the types of foods we are encouraged to consume for good health—are rich sources. When used to cure meat, nitrite gives meat like salami and ham their characteristic color and flavor and prevents the deadliest foodborne illness: botulism.

We must look at all issues in terms of a risk benefit analysis. Nitrite and nitrate, when consumed at levels found in foods, have important health effects and are even being considered as essential nutrients. For those wanting more information on this subject matter, I would recommend the book Nitrite and Nitrate in Human Health and Disease (http://www.springer.com/us/book/9783319461878).

- 9 -

Defining Nitrite and Nitrate as Nutrients

A nutrient is defined as any substance that nourishes an organism, and to nourish is to sustain with food or nutriment—to supply with what is necessary for life, health, and growth. Some categories of nutrients include water, protein, carbohydrates, vitamins, minerals, fatty acids, and amino acids. There are obviously many specific examples within each of the categories. What is clear, though, is that nutrients are fundamental to physiological systems, and proper nutrition can prevent many diseases. On the contrary, lack of nutrients can cause disease. The information already presented in this book demonstrates that nitrite and nitrate, when consumed or administered in the "right" concentrations, under the right conditions, can prevent or mitigate many diseases and improve physical performance, and therefore, classify as nutrients.

Basic science and epidemiological research have shown that all conditions of insufficient nitrite and nitrate from the diet promote or accelerate disease. To the contrary, there are many studies now showing sufficient nitrite and nitrate from dietary sources can prevent or treat many diseases and enhance physical fitness. As we advance the science of nitric oxide, it is obvious from many basic science and clinical studies that nitrite and nitrate, through the proper delivery at the right doses, have an enormous impact on many diseases that affect so many people today. Not dissimilar to vitamin K metabolism (phylloquinone or vitamin K1), nitrate serves as the primary plant form of the nutrient, whereas its metabolite nitrite is the active form (menaquinones for vitamin K) that first requires metabolic activation. The purpose of this chapter is to define the context for consideration of nitrite and nitrate as nutrients and outline optimal therapeutic levels that can easily be achieved through diet.

Origins of nitrite and nitrate

Despite historical use of inorganic nitrate and nitrite as medicinal agents—and the fact that these anions are produced naturally in the body from the oxidation of nitric oxide—along with recent demonstration of physiological roles for nitrate and nitrite in vascular and immune function, public perception is that these are harmful substances in our food and water supply. That myth was dispelled in the previous chapters. The early studies on nitrogen balance in humans demonstrated that nitrite and nitrate are synthesized de novo in the intestine. It was these early findings by Tannenbaum et al. that significantly altered our thinking about human exposure to dietary nitrite and nitrate. Prior to those studies, it was thought that steady-state levels of nitrite and nitrate in humans originated solely from the diet and from nitrogen-fixing enteric bacteria.

The endogenous production of NO from the 5-electron oxidation of L-arginine by the enzymes nitric oxide synthase (NOS) is a fundamental physiological process that maintains and regulates cardiovascular function, immune function and neurotransmission. These discoveries were so profound that the 1998 Nobel Prize in Physiology or Medicine was awarded to three U.S. scientists for the discovery of NO in the cardiovascular system. Once produced, NO has a half-life of approximately one second, and is quickly oxidized to nitrite and nitrate or reacts with amino acids on proteins. In fact, it has been shown that about 50 percent of the circulating levels of plasma nitrite reflect endogenous NO production, and steady state levels of plasma nitrite and nitrate can be affected by diet. Patients with compromised NO production from NOS, termed endothelial dysfunction, have reduced levels of plasma nitrite concentrations, and endothelial dysfunction is associated with several cardiovascular disorders. Further studies have shown that insufficient NO production is not only associated with all major cardiovascular risk factors—such as hyperlipidemia, diabetes, hypertension, smoking, and severity of atherosclerosis—but also that it has a profound predictive value for the future atherosclerotic disease progression. Therefore, steady-state levels of nitrite shown to be reflective of endogenous NO production are critical determinants of cardiovascular disease risk and progression.

Nitrite and nitrate have been used for centuries in curing and preserving meats and fish and in manufacturing certain cheeses. When added to foods, specifically meats for curing, nitrite has at least three functions. First, it contributes to the flavor due to the inhibition of the development of rancidity. Second, it reacts with myoglobin to give mononitrosylhemochrome, which forms the characteristic pink color of cured meat. Third, it inhibits the growth of food spoilage bacteria, most importantly Clostridium botulinum. C. botulinum thrives under anaerobic conditions and produces a neurotoxin that is one of the most lethal natural products known. In this regard, nitrite is critical to the food industry to prevent food borne illness from C. botulinum.

Vegetables contribute over 85 percent of the daily dietary intake of nitrate, In addition, endogenous synthesis is an important contributor to human's overall exposure of nitrate. Hord et al. estimated that approximately 80 percent of dietary nitrate is derived from vegetable consumption; therefore the primary source of exposure to nitrate by humans is through eating vegetables. Most people would not argue that a diet rich in fruits and vegetables is healthy. Recent reports have shown that less than 5 percent of the ingested nitrite and nitrate are derived from cured meat sources, with the remainder coming from vegetables and saliva.

Perhaps the most compelling argument for defining dietary nitrite and nitrate requirements comes from our knowledge on the amount of nitrite and nitrate present in breast milk of nursing mothers and their nutritional and immunological benefits to the infant. Previously published studies in our lab reveal the presence of high concentrations of nitrite and nitrate in human breast milk, consistent with previous reports. Early post-partum breast milk from certain mothers contained the highest nitrite concentration of any food or beverage product tested (near 20 µM, or 50 times higher than that found in beetroot juice). At birth, the gastrointestinal tract of the infant is sterile, and it is rapidly colonized by bacteria originating from the mother and the environment. We now know that reduction of nitrate to nitrite requires the commensal bacteria that normally reside in our body. However, in newborn infants, this pathway has not yet developed. Thus, breast milk—high in nitrite relative to nitrate—overcomes nature's deficiency early in life. At later stages of development, nitrate becomes the predominant anion when a symbiosis exists with the colonized bacteria. This becomes extremely interesting in terms of the level of nitrite exposure based on ingestion and body weight of an infant (near 1 mg/kg). Comparing these values, you begin to see discrepancy based on ignorance in terms of regulation of nitrite and nitrate exposure.

Similar to all essential or indispensable nutrients, intake of excess nitrate and nitrite exposure can be associated with increased risk of negative health outcomes, specifically low blood pressure or hypotension or methemoglobinemia (blue baby syndrome). A set of Dietary Reference Intake (DRI) categories are set by the Food and Nutrition Board of the National Academy of Sciences for essential nutrients in order to clearly define, where possible, the contexts in which intakes are deficient, safe, or potentially excessive. These DRI categories include the Recommended Dietary Allowance (RDA), Adequate Intake (AI), Tolerable Upper Level Intake (TUL), and Estimated Average Intake (EAI). The process of establishing DRIs for nutrients considers a broad range of physiological factors, not the least of which is nutritional status and potential toxicities. Such methodologies, including the consideration of normal dietary consumption patterns of nitrate- and nitrite-containing foods, have not been applied in setting exposure limits for or in considering the potential health benefits of dietary nitrate and nitrite. There are ranges for levels of intake that put people at risk of inadequacy and levels that increase the risk of excess and toxicity.

So are we at risk for being exposed to toxic levels through our diet? The National Research Council report, "The Health Effects of Nitrate, Nitrite, and N-Nitroso Compounds" (NRC 1981), estimates nitrite and nitrate intake based on food consumption tables. They report that the average total nitrite and nitrate intake in the U.S. was roughly 1 mg and 76 mg, respectively, per day. The mean intake estimates for nitrate and nitrite in the U.S. and Europe vary by investigator, but are consistent and comparable. International estimates of nitrate intakes from food are 31 to 185 mg/day in Europe and in the U.S. about 40 to 100 mg/day. The bioavailability of dietary nitrate is 100 percent. Nitrite intakes vary from 0 to 20 mg/day or up to 0.25 mg/kg body weight. Nitrate intakes from sources other than vegetables, including drinking water and cured meats, have been estimated to average 35 to 44 mg/person per day for a 60 kg human. These average intakes are much less than what is required to see any health benefits and 1000 times less than what would cause any toxicity.

Based upon a conservative recommendation to consume 400 grams of different fruits and vegetables per day at median nitrate concentrations, dietary concentration of nitrate would be ~157 mg/day. Assuming an average weight of the population to be 80kg, this equates to 1.96 mg/kg per day for nitrate. In the EU population, where fruit consumption (nitrate concentration averaging <10 mg/kg FW) constitutes over half the 400 gram intake recommendation, actual nitrate intakes would approximate 81 to 106 mg/day before additional nitrate losses are taken into account, based on washing, peeling, and/or cooking. My lab reported that persons consuming the DASH (Dietary Approaches to Stop Hypertension) diet could consume upward of 1000 mg of nitrate per day, or roughly 12.5mg/kg per day.

There are however, regulations that have been issued to prevent any toxicity. The current regulations regarding nitrite and nitrate exposure were established based on potential toxicology, primarily methemoglobinemia, and without any regard for potential health benefits. The permissible concentration of nitrate in drinking water is 50 mg nitrate per Liter (L) in the European Union (EU) and 44 mg per L in the U.S., in agreement with World Health Organization recommendations first established in 1970 and reaffirmed in 2004. The Joint Food and Agricultural Organization/World Health Organization has set the Acceptable Daily Intake (ADI) for nitrate at 3.7 mg/kg body weight and for the nitrite ion at 0.06 mg/kg body weight. The WHO ADI level for nitrate (0 to 3.7 mg/kg) translates into an equivalent of 222 mg nitrate for a 60 kg adult. The fact that typical consumption patterns of vegetables and fruit exceed regulatory limits for dietary nitrate calls into question the rationale behind current nitrate and nitrite regulations. The physiologic basis for regulating human consumption of plant foods containing nitrate and nitrite should be reevaluated to include potential health benefits.

As Paracelsus exclaimed, "Dose makes the poison." There are clear and defined doses of both nitrite and nitrate that provide indisputable evidence of promoting health and even treating serious medical conditions. Fortunately, these doses fall well below toxic and fatal doses. This provides a sufficient range for the normal dietary guidelines to be established. With such a huge difference in therapeutic and beneficial doses for nitrite and nitrate to those that are potentially toxic and harmful, this provides enough room to establish nutrient recommendations and DRIs. Until now, there has been no reason to consider an RDA for nitrite or nitrate, which is the average daily level of intake sufficient to meet the nutrient requirements of nearly all (97 to 98 percent) healthy people. Tolerable Upper Intake Level (TUL) can clearly be established, which is the maximum daily intake unlikely to cause adverse health effects.

At a time when the world is faced with epidemics of heart disease, obesity, and metabolic syndrome, we can no longer ignore fundamental nutritional, biochemical, physiological, and clinical benefits of nutrients found in the most healthy and nutritious foods—nitrite and nitrate—especially since the etiology of these diseases is based on poor diet and nutrition. As with any drug or nutrient, it is time to consider the risk benefit analysis of nitrite and nitrate. The cardiovascular benefits are clear. The risk of exposure of nitrite and nitrate and developing cancers is weak at best, but still important to consider. If we consider the WHO statistics from 2013, there were 8.2 million deaths worldwide from cancer. It is estimated that about 30 percent of cancer deaths are due to the five leading behavioral and dietary risks: high body mass index, low fruit and vegetable intake, lack of physical activity, tobacco use, and alcohol use. This would result in 2.46 million deaths from dietary and lifestyle habits, where nitrite and nitrate per se are not involved, but formation of N-nitrosamines may or may not be involved in the mechanism.

Consuming more vegetables would lead to higher intakes of nitrite and nitrate. According to WHO 2012 statistics, there were 17.3 million deaths worldwide due to cardiovascular disease, representing 30 percent of all global deaths.

Lowering blood pressure by just 5 mmHg reduces the risk of stroke by 35 percent and risk of ischemic heart disease by 21 percent, the top two killers of people worldwide. There are now clear, indisputable blood pressure lowering effects of dietary nitrite and nitrate by at least 5 mmHg. By establishing dietary guidelines for nitrite and nitrate, perhaps 35 percent—or roughly 6 million—deaths could be prevented each year. The ultimate question is how many, if any, new cases of cancers would arise from consuming an amount of nitrite and/or nitrate (that may form N-nitrosamines) to avoid cardiovascular disease. It may be impossible to determine, but we predict the cardiovascular benefits will far outweigh any risk of new cancers. It should also be highlighted that nitrite and nitrate have never been directly implicated in carcinogenesis, but only through formation of carcinogenic low molecular weight N-nitrosamines. Vitamin C and other antioxidants very effectively inhibit nitrosation reactions.

As we begin to recognize safe and effective delivery systems for nitrite and nitric oxide, we can begin to develop new technologies that will certainly have enormous benefit to human health. So, once thought as a harmful toxic molecule in our food supply, nitrite is now considered an essential nutrient and molecule produced in our body to regulate a number of physiological functions. In fact, the emerging physiological data on nitrite are strikingly analogous to a vitamin. We have referred to nitrite as a vitamin previously, and even proclaimed it "vitamin N," but perhaps it may fit the characteristics of a dietary mineral. A mineral is by definition a solid inorganic substance of natural occurrence. After all, sulfates and phosphates are recognized minerals, and nitrite and nitrate are similar in structure and composition, except replacing the sulfur and phosphorus with nitrogen respectively with different oxidation states. How we classify nitrite and nitrate may not be important at this stage other than to finally recognize them for the nutrients they are.

What we have to avoid as a scientific community and food-based companies is to begin to fortify our entire food supply with nitrite and nitrate, such as with iron or folate. In fact, beetroot bread was recently tested and found to lower diastolic blood pressure and increase endothelium-independent vasodilation. There has to be regulated and scientifically sound technologies to deliver therapeutic or dietary supplements containing nitrite and/or nitrate. The underlying chemistry of these two anions must be controlled to maximize the benefits while preventing any unwanted nitrosation chemistry causing N-nitrosamine formation. Nutritionists, physiologists, physicians, toxicologists, and dieticians need to converge and establish nutrient guidelines for nitrite and nitrate similar to other essential nutrients. The scientific evidence and facts are now available for such an initiative. Becoming more evident, is the enormous benefit of dietary nitrite and nitrate in a number of disease models. A simple ubiquitous molecule we have been advised to avoid may be an indispensable nutrient many are lacking.

- 10 -

How Much Do You Need?

It should now be clear that nitrite and nitrate from the diet can restore loss of NO production from pathway 1, the L-arginine pathway. There are many studies showing the health benefits of dietary nitrate in humans, including blood pressure regulation and sports performance. In early studies conducted in mice, relatively high doses of nitrate protected against the damaging effects of cancer chemotherapy by maintaining mitochondrial function. A much lower dose of nitrate in the drinking water of mice that cannot make nitric oxide can reverse clinical characteristics of diabetes and metabolic syndrome. For the majority of studies in humans, beetroot juice has been the dietary nitrate source of choice. However, to obtain sufficient nitrate levels for improved physical performance, a minimum of 300 to 400 mg of nitrate needs to be provided at least 2.5 hours prior to exercise in order to allow sufficient time for the uptake and metabolism of nitrate to nitrite and NO.

Research has shown that raising the nitrate and nitrite levels in the body prior to exercise by consumption of dietary nitrate can increase NO production and lead to increased oxygen efficiency and exercise performance. Additionally, in another study in older adults, dietary supplementation with beetroot juice, containing approximately 400 mg nitrate per dose twice per day (816 mg total), increased plasma nitrite concentration, reduced blood pressure, and positively influenced physiological responses to exercise. Nitrate supplementation can also enhance exercise performance in patients with peripheral artery disease. Improvements in exercise performance following beetroot juice consumption has typically been found to range between 2 to 16 percent for different types of exercise including running, cycling, rowing, and resistance exercise.

There are also several studies showing blood pressure lowering effects of nitrate when consumed through beetroot juice. Studies show that nitrate can lower blood pressure six hours later in healthy adults. Studies out of the United Kingdom had patients drink beetroot juice that contained 468 mg of nitrate and found that all forms of nitrate led to a dose dependent decrease in blood pressure beginning after ninety minutes and lasting for several hours. Similarly, other studies demonstrate that drinking beetroot juice (442 mg nitrate per day) acutely reduces blood pressure and the oxygen cost of submaximal exercise, and that these effects are maintained for at least fifteen days if supplementation is continued. Interestingly, in another study, supplementation of the diet with nitrate enriched beetroot juice for two weeks did not lower blood pressure, improve endothelial function, or improve insulin sensitivity in individuals with Type II diabetes. There appears to be patient populations that do not respond to nitrate.

Administration of roughly 500 mg nitrate for four weeks to older patients with increased cardiovascular risk profiles can reverse vascular dysfunction. There is a relatively large range of nitrate dosing that has been studied in humans and mice that provides clear therapeutic benefit without any signs of toxicity. The published studies show reductions in blood pressure of anywhere from 2 to 10 mm Hg. This change in blood pressure is very meaningful. A simple 5 mm Hg reduction in blood pressure can reduce the risk of stroke by 30 percent and the risk of heart disease by 20 percent. With 2 out of 3 Americans having high blood pressure, this approach can provide significant and profound effects on the burden of cardiovascular disease and public health.

The question then becomes, how many vegetables do I need to consume to get enough nitrite and nitrate in my diet to achieve these results? The science is very clear that one needs about 300 to 400 mg of nitrate in a single serving to achieve the positive benefits of NO in regard to blood pressure management and enhanced performance. Part of my research program set out to answer that exact question. In collaboration with the Department of Food Science at Texas A&M University, we tested five different green vegetables from five different cities across the U.S. We measured the nitrate content of broccoli, cabbage, celery, spinach, and lettuce with the intent to try to determine how many servings of each would one need to eat to get enough nitrate to reach the 300 to 400 mg needed. We went to New York, Raleigh, Dallas, Chicago, and Los Angeles and gathered these vegetables from the same retail grocer. We then took them back to the lab and analyzed them for their nitrate content. We compared conventionally grown vegetables to organically grown vegetables. What we found really surprised us. There was a greater than ten times difference in the nitrate content in specific vegetables from one city to another. Furthermore, organically grown vegetables had less nitrate than conventionally grown. The amount of nitrate in each vegetable from each city is shown in the tables below.

What this tells us is that if you lived in Dallas or Chicago, you could eat approximately 160 grams of celery and get enough nitrate from that celery to affect NO production. That is about three to four celery stalks. However, if you lived in New York or

Chicago, you would have to eat thirty to fifty stalks of celery to get a NO benefit. The same held true for spinach and lettuce as well. What about organic? We are all told that organic is better, right? Well in terms of nitrate, organically grown vegetables contain less nitrate than conventionally grown vegetables. So, organic may be better for you since they contain no herbicides or pesticides, but they do not assimilate nitrogen into nitrate, likely due to insufficient nitrogen in the soil from organic farms.

It is clear from the published clinical trials that you need 300 to 400 mg of nitrate in a single serving of vegetables to experience the benefits discussed in the previous chapters. But so is the realization that depending on where you live and what type of vegetables you are eating, people may not be getting enough nitrate from their diet. Nitrate assimilation into nitrate is dependent upon soil conditions, time of harvest, amount of fertilizer added, and water availability (drought). Historically, databases have been kept in order to keep track of how much nitrate is ingested. Based on these existing databases, the mean estimated intake for nitrate and nitrite in the U.S. and Europe varies but are consistent and somewhat comparable. International estimates of nitrate intakes from food are 31 to 185 mg/day in Europe and in the U.S. about 40 to 100 mg/day. We know from above that 300 to 400 mg in a single serving is required for NO production and improvements in blood pressure and exercise performance. Most people are consuming only half of this amount over two to three meals, and not as a single serving.

Therefore, the U.S. diet is depleted in nitrate. As a result, Americans are a nitrate deficient society. The research suggests that this deficiency may be partly responsible for the increased incidence of all cardiovascular related diseases in the U.S. population. Consistent with this notion, certain diets provide much more nitrate. For example, the Dietary Approaches to Stop Hypertension (DASH) diet can provide as much as 1200 mg nitrate per day from choosing certain foods. The Japanese diet also provides more than 500 mg nitrate that has been shown to reduce blood pressure and improve performance. Similarly, the Mediterranean diet provides sufficient nitrate along with antioxidants to support reduction of nitrate to nitrite and nitric oxide. There is strong evidence that it is the dietary nitrate and nitrite in these foods and diets that confer the protective and health promoting activities. Although many clinical trials have been performed to try to identify the mechanism of action of these diets, looking primarily at antioxidants, vitamins, and minerals, most have failed to recapitulate the effects of the whole food diets.

Evidence strongly suggests that it is the nitrate/nitrite content along with the antioxidants that account for the effects. However, it is not as simple as we would hope. Nitrate itself is inactive and without effect. Nitrate must first be reduced by oral commensal bacteria to nitrite, and then nitrite has biological activity. As described above, only about 5 percent of the total nitrate is reduced to nitrite. All biological effects of nitrate are abolished by antiseptic mouthwash that kills oral bacteria. The next chapter will reveal how to best utilize functional nitric oxide nutrition to restore NO production.

Mean nitrate (NO_3^-) concentrations (mg/kg) of raw vegetables classified as conventional from each city

Product category	Chicago	Dallas	Los Angeles	New York	Raleigh
Broccoli	271 ± 89	357 ± 50	512 ± 85	279 ± 80	553 ± 28
Cabbage	475 ± 46	256 ± 33	800 ± 142	193 ± 28	364 ± 79
Celery	230 ± 19	2052 ± 156	2651 ± 339	88 ± 17	2201 ± 112
Lettuce	207 ± 32	1370 ± 93	1051 ± 122	568 ± 93	986 ± 185
Spinach	647 ± 69	4923 ± 327	4138 ± 451	564 ± 174	3155 ± 145

FUNCTIONAL NITRIC OXIDE NUTRITION

Mean nitrate (NO_3^-) concentrations (mg/kg) of raw vegetables classified as organic from each city

Product category	Chicago	Dallas	Los Angeles	New York	Raleigh
Broccoli	212 ± 35	430 ± 40	196 ± 47	167 ± 53	8 ± 2
Cabbage	53 ± 12	989 ± 166	612 ± 85	898 ± 191	167 ± 18
Celery	310 ± 58	390 ± 139	2022 ± 208	807 ± 208	1023 ± 69
Lettuce	100 ± 8	1367 ± 99	1277 ± 73	780 ± 111	692 ± 28
Spinach	459 ± 48	1610 ± 209	2199 ± 237	1566 ± 384	755 ± 101

- 11 -

Now What? Simple Steps to Regain your Health

The benefits of dietary nitrite and nitrate are indisputable. The amount you need to see drastic improvements in health and wellness are far below levels that would cause any concern for toxicity or harmful effects. Even if we consume sufficient nitrate from our diet, if it is not first metabolized and reduced to nitrite, the human body cannot utilize it to make nitric oxide. Humans do not have a functional nitrate reductase gene. As we have learned from earlier chapters, this metabolism is dependent upon oral bacteria. Nitrate ingested from the diet is rapidly absorbed in the small intestine, taken up into circulation where it mixes with the endogenous nitrate from oxidation of nitric oxide, and readily distributed throughout the body. About 25 percent of oral nitrate from diet is concentrated and excreted by salivary glands, so that salivary nitrate concentration is approximately ten times higher in the saliva than in plasma. Approximately 20 percent of salivary nitrate can be reduced to nitrite in the mouth by facultative anaerobic bacteria, which are found on the dorsal surface of the tongue if nitrate-reducing bacteria are present, resulting in about a 5 percent reduction of total ingested nitrate to nitrite.

If we are consuming 300 to 400 mg nitrate from our diet, which is the dose known to be effective at reducing blood pressure and enhancing performance, then this reduction efficacy results in 15 to 20 mg nitrite produced from dietary nitrate through the enterosalivary circuit. Nitrate, when consumed through the diet, reaches peak blood levels in about an hour. The levels will remain elevated for about five to six hours. The high concentration of nitrate and nitrite in saliva and other tissue, continuous production from nitric oxide, and the re-absorption from renal tubules strongly suggest that nitrate and nitrite have a definite role in normal human physiology and are not just unwanted toxins. They serve as important substrates for NO production, provided the body can utilize them.

So how can you optimize your nitric oxide production? As mentioned earlier, the evidence suggests that the U.S. diet is deficient in nitrate. Furthermore, common drug therapy and lifestyle decisions disrupt metabolism of nitrate into nitrite and nitric oxide. So, people taking antibiotics, antiseptic mouthwash, and/or antacid drugs further disrupt the benefits of getting nitrate from the diet. How does one overcome deficiencies in dietary nitrate, variability between individual microbiomes, mouthwash use, PPI use, or insufficient stomach acid production? We and others have focused on nitrite. Nitrite is the metabolic product of nitrate reduction by the bacteria. Nitrite itself can be utilized by human enzyme systems to generate and produce NO, and is not dependent upon oral bacteria. Nitrite is derived directly from exogenous dietary nitrate, but also from the oxidation of endogenously produced nitric oxide. Nitrite is found naturally in colostrum and breast milk, small amounts found naturally in green leafy vegetables, and small amounts added to cured meats.

Whereas daily nitrate intakes vary from 150 to 300 mg from the diet, nitrite intake from food varies from 5 to 40 mg/day.

When we measure actual NO production in young healthy adults, this varies between 0.15 and 2.2 μmol/kg/hour. When we convert this production rate to the amount of nitrite this produces as a consequence of sufficient NO production, for a 150- to 170-pound person this would equate to approximately 20 to 200 mg nitrite and nitrate daily. Due to approximately 5 percent reduction of nitrate (average of 150 mg per day in U.S. diet plus 200 mg from oxidation of NO), this would equate to 17.5 mg endogenous nitrite production. Therefore, total daily nitrite exposure in a normal healthy individual on a Western diet is roughly 20 to 40 mg. For the same healthy individual consuming more of a vegetarian diet or DASH diet that included 400 to 1200 mg nitrate per day, endogenous nitrite production could exceed 70 mg per day. These nitrite levels are dramatically reduced in people with endothelial dysfunction, insufficient vegetable consumption, or consuming vegetables without sufficient nitrate along with use of antibiotics/antiseptic mouthwash and/or PPIs.

These data beg the question that if most people are nitrite deficient, can we safely and adequately supplement back what is missing? This approach is no different than vitamin D, for example. If labs demonstrate we are low in vitamin D, then you supplement what is missing in order to normalize your levels. This has been our approach with nitrite and nitrate.

There are a number of published studies in humans showing the safety and efficacy of nitrite within a large range of doses. Sodium nitrite capsules at doses of 160 mg and 320 mg were used to determine toxicity and pharmacokinetics. Nitrite even at a dose of 320 mg did not show any clinically toxic levels of methemoglobinemia (<15 percent). However, some subjects reported mild headache and nausea that resolved after a half-hour. This study also revealed that nitrite is 98 percent orally available. Another study using a sodium nitrite capsule in diabetics demonstrated that a single administration of 80 mg sodium nitrite was well tolerated with no significant changes in any measures of toxicity. The 80 mg nitrite dose led to a significant drop in systolic blood pressure with no effect on diastolic pressures.

Chronic studies using 80 to 160 mg nitrite capsules for ten weeks in a randomized, placebo-control, double-blind study increased plasma nitrite acutely and chronically and was well tolerated without an unsafe drop in blood pressure. Endothelial function, measured by brachial artery flow-mediated dilation, was significantly improved without changes in body mass or blood lipids. Carotid artery elasticity (as measured by ultrasound and applanation tonometry) improved. These functional changes were related to eleven specific metabolites that could predict the vascular changes with nitrite. Similarly, in another study using 80 and 160 mg nitrite capsules for ten weeks showed improvement in performance on measures of motor and cognitive outcomes in healthy middle aged and older adults (62 ± 7 years). These studies provide evidence that sodium nitrite supplementation is well tolerated, increases plasma nitrite concentrations, improves endothelial function, lessens carotid artery stiffening, and improves motor and cognitive function in middle-aged and older adults, perhaps by altering multiple metabolic pathways. The effects of nitrite are not dependent upon oral nitrate-reducing bacteria, and appear to be safe even at doses that far exceed daily human production.

Sodium nitrite also appears to have a positive effect in compromised patients. In a double-blind, randomized, placebo-controlled, parallel-group trial, subjects with heart failure with preserved ejection fraction (HFpEF) underwent invasive cardiac catheterization with simultaneous expired gas analysis at rest and during exercise, before and fifteen minutes after treatment with either sodium nitrite or a matching placebo. Before the nitrite infusion, HFpEF subjects displayed an increase in pulmonary capillary wedge pressure (PCWP) with exercise from 16 ± 5 mm Hg to 30 ± 7 mm Hg (p < 0.0001). After nitrite infusion, the primary endpoint of exercise PCWP was substantially improved by nitrite compared with the placebo (adjusted mean: 19 ± 5 mm Hg vs. 28 ± 6 mm Hg; p = 0.0003). Nitrite-enhanced cardiac output reserve improved with exercise and normalized the increase in cardiac output relative to oxygen consumption. Nitrite improved pulmonary artery pressure-flow relationships in HFpEF and increased left ventricular stroke work with exercise versus placebo, indicating an improvement in ventricular performance with stress (Borlaug et al. 2015). These authors conclude that acute sodium nitrite infusion favorably attenuates hemodynamic derangements of cardiac failure that develop during exercise in individuals with HFpEF.

The doses of nitrite used in these studies are typically more than one would normally consume in an ordinary diet. This is in part due to the fact that nitrite is inefficiently reduced to NO along the physiological oxygen gradient, and therefore more is needed to get any appreciable amount of NO produced—especially in people who are NO deficient. Through the discovery of natural product chemistry of an oxygen independent nitrite reductase, lower supplemental doses of nitrite can more effectively reduce nitrite to NO and therefore provide an exogenous source of NO in the oral cavity. The premise of this technology is that if your body can't make NO due to endothelial dysfunction, oral dysbiosis, antiseptic mouthwash, or PPI use, then this will provide an exogenous source of NO.

Studies using a patented composition of matter formulation (Neo40™, HumanN, Inc™)—with a standardized amount of nitrite along with a functional nitrite reductase for the generation of NO to account for differences in endogenous production along with the natural product chemistry in the form of an orally disintegrating tablet—found that nitrite could modify cardiovascular risk factors in patients over the age of 40, significantly reduce triglycerides, and reduce blood pressure. Single administration of this lozenge leads to peak plasma levels of nitrite around 1.5 µM. In patients with argininosuccinic aciduria (ASA), the nitrite lozenge led to a significant reduction in blood pressure when prescription medications were ineffective, improved renal function and cognition, and reversed cardiac hypertrophy. Another randomized controlled study using the nitrite lozenge showed that a single lozenge can significantly reduce blood pressure, dilate blood vessels, and improve endothelial function and arterial compliance in hypertensive patients. Furthermore, in a study of pre-hypertensive patients (BP >120/80 < 139/89), administration of one lozenge twice daily leads to a significant reduction in blood pressure (12 mmHg systolic and 6 mmHg diastolic) after thirty days, along with improvements in functional capacity as measured by a six-minute walk test. In an exercise study, the nitrite lozenge significantly improved exercise performance.

Most recently, in subjects with stable carotid plaque, the NO lozenge led to a 11 percent reduction in carotid plaque after six months. To put this in perspective, meta-analysis of trials using treatment with statins (cholesterol-lowering medication) reported that a total of seven trials showed regression and four trials showed slowing of progression of CIMT of approximately 2.7 percent (-0.04) after more than two years. Using the nitric oxide lozenge, the data show an average of 0.073 mm or 10.9 percent after six months. Similarly, this same patented technology in the form of a concentrated beetroot powder (Superbeets™, HumanN, Inc.™) attenuates peripheral chemoreflex sensitivity without concomitant change in spontaneous cardiovagal baroreflex sensitivity, while also reducing systemic blood pressure and mean arterial blood pressure in older adults. These studies clearly demonstrate the safety and efficacy of low supplemental doses of nitrite in humans that can correct for any insufficiencies from dietary exposure, pharmacological inhibition by antiseptics, or PPIs.

Is this what nature intended?

If supplementing deficient nitrite and nitrate in populations is a viable strategy for combatting cardiovascular disease or any condition associated with insufficient nitric oxide availability, are there examples in the epidemiology literature with specific populations that can provide justification for such? The answer may come in the form of nature's most perfect food, breast milk. We and others have published analyses showing that early breast milk and colostrum contain high concentrations of nitrite until the bacteria begin to colonize in the oral and digestive tract of growing infants. Once commensal bacteria have colonized, breast milk changes from nitrite to nitrate so that the infant's body can utilize the nitrate-reducing bacteria to provide a more extended exposure to nitrite. Commercial infant formulas lack any nitrite and have very little nitrate. The health disparities between breastfed and formula-fed babies are well known. Supplementing nitrite that is missing in formula can protect from necrotizing enterocolitis.

Additionally, anthropological studies on native Tibetans reveal that their acclimatization to living at high altitude and reduced oxygen is through increased nitric oxide production with 20 to 50 times higher circulating nitrite and nitrate than those who live at sea level. People who live at or near sea level increase their NO production and plasma levels of nitrite and nitrate as they ascend to altitude. Increasing nitrite and nitrate availability is a physiological response to low oxygen, and the adaptive response to allow us to acclimate to different environments. In other words, increasing steady state concentrations of nitrite and nitrate appears to be a natural physiological response that allows the body to adapt to changing oxygen environments, whether environmental or physiological.

To summarize, there are really some simple steps you can take to ensure sufficient and adequate nitric oxide production to maintain healthy circulation, blood flow, and cellular function.

If you follow the steps below you can allow your body to make NO and be in the best health you can be.

1. Eat more green leafy vegetables.

2. Get moderate physical exercise (twenty minutes, three to five times per week).

3. Stop using antiseptic mouthwash and do not overuse antibiotics.

4. Stop using antacids. You need stomach acid to make NO.

5. Supplement your diet with standardized nitric oxide functional nutrition products.

The next question is, how do you know what standardized nitric oxide functional nutrition products are? There are many nitric oxide products on the market. When searching for a "functional" nitric oxide product, look for four things:

1. Are there any published clinical trials conducted on the actual product? Clinical trials are expensive to conduct, and most dietary supplements are not rigorously studied in clinical trials.

2. Are there any patents listed on the product label? Patents or licenses from universities or medical schools demonstrate that the product is innovative and unlike any other product on the market.

3. Is the product from a reputable company that is focused on nitric oxide innovations? There are many reputable companies that make good products that aren't related to nitric oxide. NO is a complicated science and requires expertise and know how. If the company isn't experienced in NO, then their products will typically not work.

4. Has the inventor or formulator of the product ever published in the nitric oxide field? Many people can put ingredients together, but one must be experienced in nitric oxide research. Peer-reviewed publications are a great metric for determining if the company or formulator is an expert in nitric oxide.

These are simple steps to make sure you find and take products that work. Functional nitric oxide nutrition may be the most important consideration for your health and wellness. The published science tells us that your body cannot and will not heal or perform optimally without fixing the dysfunction nitric oxide production pathways. I trust the information in this book will provide you with the information and knowledge to help you make decisions that will improve your health.

- 12 -

Looking Forward

Regular intake of nitrate- and nitrite-containing foods may ensure that blood and tissue levels of nitrite and NO pools are maintained at a level sufficient to compensate for any disturbances in endogenous NO synthesis from NOS. Since low levels of supplemental nitrite and nitrate have been shown to enhance blood flow, dietary sources of NO metabolites can, therefore, improve blood flow and oxygen delivery, and protect against various cardiovascular disease states or any condition associated with NO insufficiency. As science advances and new discoveries and understandings are made, it is important to be able to incorporate these new findings into meaningful guidelines that can enhance health, lengthen life, and reduce illness and disability. Translating new science discoveries to medical practice or public health policy takes approximately seventeen years, which is way too long for the health benefits to be realized.

We now know that "Dose makes the poison." Fortunately the doses of both nitrite and nitrate that are effective at lowering blood pressure, improving circulation and performance are about 100 times less than what would cause any toxicity. Furthermore, the safe and efficacious doses can be obtained from foods and standardized supplements. Amounts found naturally in food will never reach levels of toxicity. The science has shown clearly that a healthy diet should not only focus on reducing sugar and caloric intake, but on adding foodstuffs promoting nitric oxide bioactivity, which can include foods enriched in nitrite, nitrate, L-arginine, and antioxidants to promote NO production and availability. This pathway is also the current focus of a number of biotechnology and pharmaceutical companies in their attempts to develop NO- and nitrite-based therapeutics.

In 2016, total healthcare expenditures in the U.S. exceeded $3.3 trillion up 4% from the previous year, or $10,348 per person, accounting for almost 18% of the Gross Domestic Product (GDP). This trend is expected to increase over the coming years, increasing by 5.6% every year for the next ten years. Currently, costs associated with chronic diseases such as obesity, diabetes, hypertension, coronary artery disease account for 75 percent of the nation's annual healthcare costs. According to the American Heart Association, an estimated 92 million people had one or more forms of cardiovascular disease in the U.S. in 2016, (up 12% from a 2006) including hypertension, coronary artery disease, myocardial infarction, angina pectoris, stroke, and heart failure. By 2030, 43.9% of the US adult population is projected to have some form of CVD. Most, if not all, chronic diseases that lead to the highly prevalent burden of cardiovascular disorders, including diabetes and obesity, are the result of a dysfunctional endothelium and inability to produce NO and/or maintain NO homeostasis and signaling. Understanding and developing new strategies to restore NO homeostasis will have a profound impact on public health and on the health care system. Defining the context for the role of nitrite and nitrate in human health and disease is an essential first step in the process.

We are at the beginning of a new field in nutritional biochemistry as it relates to nitrite and nitrate. Historically, we have relied on databases for average nitrite and nitrate content of certain and specifics foods. Then, based on food frequency questionnaires, we are able to assess a daily exposure value for both nitrite and nitrate. Our most recent survey of both vegetables and cured and processed meats report very large differences in nitrite and nitrate content of certain meats and vegetables, but also regional differences as well as differences between conventional versus organically grown vegetables. In fact, there exists as much as a thirty-fold difference between conventional nitrate content of conventionally grown celery between cities, and as much as a fifty-four-fold difference in organically grown broccoli between cities. This presents obvious problems with using food frequency questionnaires and dated databases for estimations of nitrite and nitrate exposure. The variation in compositional content, specifically nitrate concentration, of organically and conventionally produced raw vegetables (highly consumed) may need to be considered when compiling nutrient composition databases. If compositional differences are of sufficient magnitude, this might warrant an "organic" category in databases to be an additional factor to consider when modeling nutrient intake. For epidemiological studies investigating nitrite and nitrate exposure, it will be necessary to obtain and measure the actual foods consumed in order to get an accurate value for individual exposures. Furthermore, long-term controlled studies need to be conducted to establish set amounts of nitrite and/or nitrate consumption to determine if certain doses can actually have an effect on the onset and/or progression of chronic disease in humans. The only way to do this is through functional nitric oxide nutrition with standardized amounts of nitrite and nitrate in foods and supplements.

The most reasonable conclusion that can be made from the data reviewed is that humans are adapted to receive dietary nitrite and nitrate from birth and throughout life, and therefore nitrite and nitrate may not pose significant risks at levels naturally found in certain foods. In fact, we believe the absence of these essential nutrients in our diets may be involved in many of the chronic health problems facing the entire developing world. Advancements in science and research over the past thirty years have illuminated the essential nature of nitrite and nitrate in our food supply as well as how our body makes these natural molecules. Eating a well-balanced, nutritious diet and performing moderate exercise comprise the ideal model of routinely good health and disease prevention. The role of a proper diet in the prevention of disease is well established by many population-based epidemiological studies. Nothing affects our health more than what we choose to eat.

Nitric oxide is essential for maintaining normal blood pressure, preventing adhesion of blood cells to the endothelium, and preventing platelet aggregation; it may, therefore, be argued that this single abnormality, the inability to generate NO, puts us at risk for diseases that plague us later in life. Developing strategies and new technologies designed to restore NO availability is essential for inhibiting the progression of these common chronic diseases. The provision of dietary nitrate and nitrite may allow for such a strategy. In fact, understanding how the body utilizes key dietary nutrients, specifically nitrate, will help scientists and physicians develop more effective treatment strategies for overcoming key limitations in our diet or metabolism of dietary constituents. Indeed, implementing functional nitric oxide nutrition has the potential to profoundly change the face of health and disease.

About the Author

Dr. Bryan earned his undergraduate Bachelor of Science degree in Biochemistry from the University of Texas at Austin, and his doctoral degree from Louisiana State University School of Medicine in Shreveport, where he was the recipient of the Dean's Award for Excellence in Research. He pursued his post-doctoral training as a Kirschstein Fellow at Boston University School of Medicine in the Whitaker Cardiovascular Institute. After a two-year post-doctoral fellowship, in 2006 Dr. Bryan was recruited to join faculty at the University of Texas Health Science Center at Houston by Ferid Murad, M.D., Ph.D., 1998 Nobel Laureate in Medicine or Physiology.

During his tenure as faculty and independent investigator at UT, his research focused on drug discovery through screening natural product libraries for active compounds. His nine years at UT led to several discoveries, which have resulted in more than a dozen issued US and international patents and many more pending. Specifically, Dr. Bryan was the first to describe nitrite and nitrate as indispensable nutrients required for optimal cardiovascular health. He was the first to demonstrate and discover an endocrine function of nitric oxide via the formation of S-nitrosoglutathione and inorganic nitrite. Through the drug discovery program in natural product chemistry, Dr. Bryan discovered unique compositions of matter that can be used to safely and effectively generate and restore nitric oxide in humans. This technology is now validated in multiple published clinical trials.

Dr. Bryan is also a successful entrepreneur who has commercialized his nitric oxide technology through the formation and Founding of a University of Texas Health Science Center portfolio company, named to the Inc 5000 fastest growing companies in the US for many years ongoing.

Dr. Bryan has been involved in nitric oxide research for several decades and has made many seminal discoveries in the field. These discoveries and findings have transformed the development of safe and effective functional bioactive natural products in the treatment and prevention of human disease and may provide the basis for new preventive or therapeutic strategies in many chronic diseases. Dr. Bryan has published a number of highly cited papers and authored or edited 5 books. He is an international leader in molecular medicine and nitric oxide biochemistry. He is also a rancher raising registered Hereford cattle. In his free time, Dr. Bryan enjoys golfing and roping.

About Dr. Bryan's Work

Dr. Bryan has spent his entire professional career researching nitric oxide. His research program has always been very focused on two main objectives:

1. To understand what goes wrong in people who can't make nitric oxide.

2. Identify nutritional and therapeutic strategies to fix the underlying biochemistry and physiology to restore normal NO production.

This endeavor has resulted in discoveries that have the potential to change the management and prevention of chronic disease. Loss of nitric oxide is the earliest event in the onset and progression of most, if not all, chronic diseases. Understanding how to fix the underlying problem of NO insufficiency will transform public health and disease management.

His current research projects include identification and characterization of oral nitrate reducing bacteria that provide the human host with a continuous source of nitrite and nitric oxide. Lack of these oral bacteria leads to chronic NO deficiency and all that entails, including increase in blood pressure, exercise intolerance, poor circulation, and loss of nitric oxide-based signaling. This new paradigm then focuses on the oral microbiome as a therapeutic target to manage blood pressure and nitric oxide-based functions.

Restoring nitric oxide production in the human body is essential for humans to perform to their full potential and prevent age-related disease. Your body cannot and will not heal until you fix the nitric oxide production pathways.

Other Books by Dr. Bryan

Beet the Odds: Harness the Power of Beets to Radically Transform Your Health by Nathan S. Bryan, PhD, Carolyn Pierini, CLS (ASCP), CNC – Neogenis Laboratories 2013

Food, Nutrition and the Nitric Oxide Pathway: Biochemistry and Bioactivity by Nathan S. Bryan, PhD - DesTech Publications, Inc. 2010

Nitrite and Nitrate in Human Health and Disease by Nathan S. Bryan, Joseph Loscalzo – Humana Press 2011

The Nitric Oxide (NO) Solution: How to Boost the Body's Miracle Molecule to Prevent and Reverse Chronic Disease by Nathan S. Bryan, PhD, Janet Zand, OMD, with Bill Gottlieb, CHC – Neogenis Labs 2010

Connect with the Author

Website: www.drnathansbryan.com

Email: drnathanbryan@gmail.com

Social Media:

Facebook:
https://www.facebook.com/nathan.bryan.16

LinkedIn:
https://www.linkedin.com/in/nathan-bryan-27586b7/

Twitter: @drnathanbryan

Acknowledgements

I have had many mentors, teachers, and colleagues that have inspired me to ask the tough questions, design good experiments, and recognize all scientific observations are meaningful even if it was not what was expected. These include my first mentor, Martin Feelisch, Ph.D, good friend and colleague Tienush Rassaf, M.D., Ph.D., friend and co-author on a previous book Joseph Loscalzo, M.D., Ph.D., and Ferid Murad, M.D., Ph.D., who hired me for my first faculty position. David Lefer, Ph.D., who mentored me and collaborated with me as I established my research program. John P. Cooke, M.D., Ph.D., who is someone I have always looked up to and respected in the NO field. C. Thomas Caskey, M.D., for believing in my science and encouragement early on in my commercial ventures. Last but certainly not least, my family for their unending support and encouragement even during my many nights away from home.

References

Aisaka, K., et al. "L-arginine availability determines the duration of acetylcholine-induced systemic vasodilation in vivo." *Biochem Biophys Res Commun* 163, no. 2 (1989): 710-7.

Amaral, J.H., et al. "TEMPOL enhances the antihypertensive effects of sodium nitrite by mechanisms facilitating nitrite-derived gastric nitric oxide formation." *Free Radic Biol Med* 65 (2013): 446-55.

Arnold, W.P., et al. "Nitric oxide activates guanylate cyclase and increases guanosine 3':5'-cyclic monophosphate levels in various tissue preparations." *Proc Natl Acad Sci USA* 74, no. 8 (1977): 3203-7.

Bailey, S.J., et al. "Dietary nitrate supplementation enhances muscle contractile efficiency during knee-extensor exercise in humans." *J Appl Physiol* 109, no. 1 (2010): 135-48.

Bedi, U.S., et al. "Effects of statins on progression of carotid atherosclerosis as measured by carotid intimal--medial thickness: a meta-analysis of randomized controlled trials." *J Cardiovasc Pharmacol Ther* 15, no. 3 (2010): 268-73.

Berkowitz, D.E., et al. "Arginase reciprocally regulates nitric oxide synthase activity and contributes to endothelial dysfunction in aging blood vessels." *Circulation* 108, no. 16 (2003): 2000-6.

Biswas, O.S., V.R. Gonzalez, and E.R. Schwarz. "Effects of an Oral Nitric Oxide Supplement on Functional Capacity and Blood Pressure in Adults With Prehypertension." *J Cardiovasc Pharmacol Ther* (2014).

Blair, S.N., et al. "Physical fitness and all-cause mortality. A prospective study of healthy men and women." *JAMA* 262, no. 17 (1989): 2395-401.

Bock, J.M., et al. "Inorganic nitrate supplementation attenuates peripheral chemoreflex sensitivity but does not improve cardiovagal baroreflex sensitivity in older adults." *Am J Physiol Heart Circ Physiol* (2017): ajpheart 00389 2017.

Boolell, M., et al. "Sildenafil: an orally active type 5 cyclic GMP-specific phosphodiesterase inhibitor for the treatment of penile erectile dysfunction." *Int J Impot Res* 8, no. 2 (1996): 47-52.

Bryan, N.S., and H. Van Grinsven. "The Role of Nitrate in Human Health." In *Advances in Agronomy*, edited by D.L. Sparks, 153-76. New York: Elsevier, 2013.

Bryan, N.S., and J.L. Ivy. "Inorganic nitrite and nitrate: evidence to support consideration as dietary nutrients." *Nutr Res* 35, no. 8 (2015): 643-54.

Bryan, N.S., and J. Loscalzo, eds. *Nitrite and Nitrate in Human Health and Disease.* New York: Humana Press, 2011.

Bryan, N.S., et al. "Nitrite is a signaling molecule and regulator of gene expression in mammalian tissues." *Nat Chem Biol* 1, no. 5 (2005): 290-7.

Bryan, N.S., K. Bian, and F. Murad. "Discovery of the nitric oxide signaling pathway and targets for drug development." *Front Biosci* 14 (2009): 1-18.

Bryan, N.S. "Nitrite in nitric oxide biology: Cause or consequence? A systems-based review." *Free Radic Biol Med* 41, no. 5 (2006): 691-701.

Cekmen, M.B., et al. "Decreased adrenomedullin and total nitrite levels in breast milk of preeclamptic women." *Clin Biochem* 37, no. 2 (2004): 146-8.

Coles, L.T., and P.M. Clifton. "Effect of beetroot juice on lowering blood pressure in free-living, disease-free adults: a randomized, placebo-controlled trial." *Nutr J* 11 (2012): 106.

Cooke, J.P., and Y.T. Ghebremariam. "DDAH says NO to ADMA." *Arterioscler Thromb Vasc Biol* 31, no. 7 (2011): 1462-4.

Cooper, K.H., et al. "Physical fitness levels vs selected coronary risk factors. A cross-sectional study." *JAMA* 236, no. 2 (1976): 166-9.

Cosby, K., et al. "Nitrite reduction to nitric oxide by deoxyhemoglobin vasodilates the human circulation." *Nature Medicine* 9 (2003): 1498-1505.

Cutler, J.A., et al. "Trends in hypertension prevalence, awareness, treatment, and control rates in United States adults between 1988-1994 and 1999-2004." *Hypertension* 52, no. 5 (2008): 818-27.

Dayoub, H., et al. "Dimethylarginine dimethylaminohydrolase regulates nitric oxide synthesis: genetic and physiological evidence." *Circulation* 108, no. 24 (2003): 3042-7.

DeVan, A.E., et al. "Effects of sodium nitrite supplementation on vascular function and related small metabolite signatures in middle-aged and older adults." *J Appl Physiol* (2015): jap 00879 2015.

Doel, J.J., et al. "Evaluation of bacterial nitrate reduction in the human oral cavity." *Eur J Oral Sci* 113, no. 1 (2005): 14-9.

Egashira, K., et al. "Effects of age on endothelium-dependent vasodilation of resistance coronary artery by acetylcholine in humans." *Circulation* 88, no. 1 (1993): 77-81.

Erez, A., et al. "Requirement of argininosuccinate lyase for systemic nitric oxide production." *Nat Med* 17, no. 12 (2011): 1619-26.

Erzurum, S.C., et al. "Higher blood flow and circulating NO products offset high-altitude hypoxia among Tibetans." *Proc Natl Acad Sci USA* 104, no. 45 (2007): 17593-8.

Feelisch, M., et al. "Tissue Processing of Nitrite in Hypoxia: An Intricate Interplay of Nitric Oxide -Generating and - Scavenging Systems." *J Biol Chem* 283, no. 49 (2008): 33927-34.

Fleming-Dutra, K.E., et al. "Prevalence of Inappropriate Antibiotic Prescriptions Among US Ambulatory Care Visits, 2010-2011." *JAMA* 315, no. 17 (2016): 1864-73.

Gangolli, S.D., et al. "Nitrate, nitrite and N-nitroso compounds." *Eur J Pharmacol* 292, no. 1 (1994): 1-38.

Gerhard, M., et al. "Aging progressively impairs endothelium-dependent vasodilation in forearm resistance vessels of humans." *Hypertension* 27, no. 4 (1996): 849-53.

Ghebremariam, Y.T., et al. "Unexpected effect of proton pump inhibitors: elevation of the cardiovascular risk factor asymmetric dimethylarginine." *Circulation* 128, no. 8 (2013): 845-53.

Godfrey, M., and D.S. Majid. "Renal handling of circulating nitrates in anesthetized dogs." *Am J Physiol* 275 (1998): F68-73.

Govoni, M., et al. "The increase in plasma nitrite after a dietary nitrate load is markedly attenuated by an antibacterial mouthwash." *Nitric Oxide* 19, no. 4 (2008): 333-7.

Green, D.J., et al. "Control of skeletal muscle blood flow during dynamic exercise: contribution of endothelium-derived nitric oxide." *Sports Med* 21, no. 2 (1996): 119-46.

Green, L.C., et al. "Nitrate biosynthesis in man." *Proc Natl Acad Sci USA* 78, no. 12 (1981): 7764-8.

Greenway, F.L., et al. "Single-dose pharmacokinetics of different oral sodium nitrite formulations in diabetes patients." *Diabetes Technol Ther* 14, no. 7 (2012): 552-60.

Hecker, M., et al. "Endothelial cells metabolize NG-monomethyl-L-arginine to L-citrulline and subsequently to

L-arginine." *Biochem Biophys Res Commun* 167, no. 3 (1990): 1037-43.

Hibbs, J.B., Jr., R.R. Taintor, and Z. Vavrin. "Macrophage cytotoxicity: role for L-arginine deiminase and imino nitrogen oxidation to nitrite." *Science* 235, no. 4787 (1987): 473-6.

Hord, N.G., et al. "Nitrate and nitrite content of human, formula, bovine, and soy milks: implications for dietary nitrite and nitrate recommendations." *Breastfeed Med* 6, no. 6 (2011): 393-9.

Hord, N.G., Y. Tang, and N.S. Bryan. "Food sources of nitrates and nitrites: the physiologic context for potential health benefits." *Am J Clin Nutr* 90, no. 1 (2009): 1-10.

Houston, M., and L. Hays. "Acute effects of an oral nitric oxide supplement on blood pressure, endothelial function, and vascular compliance in hypertensive patients." *J Clin Hypertens (Greenwich)* 16, no. 7 (2014): 524-9.

Hunault, C.C., et al. "Bioavailability of sodium nitrite from an aqueous solution in healthy adults." *Toxicol Lett* 190, no. 1 (2009): 48-53.

Hyde, E.R., et al. "Metagenomic analysis of nitrate-reducing bacteria in the oral cavity: implications for nitric oxide homeostasis." *PLoS One* 9, no. 3 (2014): e88645.

Justice, J.N., et al. "Improved motor and cognitive performance with sodium nitrite supplementation is related to small metabolite signatures: a pilot trial in middle-aged and older adults." *Aging* 7, no. 11 (2015): 1004-21.

Kannel, W.B., T. Gordon, and M.J. Schwartz. "Systolic versus diastolic blood pressure and risk of coronary heart disease. The Framingham study." *Am J Cardiol* 27, no. 4 (1971): 335-46.

Kapil, V., et al. "Inorganic nitrate supplementation lowers blood pressure in humans: role for nitrite-derived NO." *Hypertension* 56, no. 2 (2010): 274-81.

Kapil, V., et al. "Physiological role for nitrate-reducing oral bacteria in blood pressure control." *Free Radic Biol Med* 55 (2013): 93-100.

Kelly, J., et al. "Effects of short-term dietary nitrate supplementation on blood pressure, O2 uptake kinetics, and muscle and cognitive function in older adults." *Am J Physiol Regul Integr Comp Physiol* 304, no. 2 (2013): R73-83.

Kelm, M. "Nitric oxide metabolism and breakdown." *Biochimica et Biophysica Acta* 1411 (1999): 273-289.

Kenjale, A.A., et al. "Dietary nitrate supplementation enhances exercise performance in peripheral arterial disease." *J Appl Physiol* 110, no. 6 (1985): 1582-91.

Kevil, C.G., et al. "Inorganic nitrite therapy: historical perspective and future directions." *Free Radic Biol Med* 51, no. 3 (2011): 576-93.

Kleinbongard, P., et al. "Plasma nitrite reflects constitutive nitric oxide synthase activity in mammals." *Free Radical Biology & Medicine* 35, no. 7 (2003): 790-796.

Lakatta, E.G., and F.C. Yin. "Myocardial aging: functional alterations and related cellular mechanisms." *Am J Physiol* 242, no. 6 (1982): H927-41.

Landmesser, U., et al. "Oxidation of tetrahydrobiopterin leads to uncoupling of endothelial cell nitric oxide synthase in hypertension." *J Clin Invest* 111, no. 8 (2003): 1201-9.

Lansley, K.E., et al. "Dietary nitrate supplementation reduces the O2 cost of walking and running: a placebo-controlled study." *J Appl Physiol* 110, no. 3 (2011): 591-600.

Larsen, F.J., et al. "Effects of dietary nitrate on blood pressure in healthy volunteers." *N Engl J Med* 355, no. 26 (2006): 2792-3.

Lee, E. "Effects of Nitric Oxide on Carotid Intima Media Thickness: A Pilot Study." *Alternative Therapies in Health and Medicine* 22, no. 2 (2016): 32-34.

Lee, J., et al. "Caffeinated Nitric Oxide-releasing Lozenge Improves Cycling Time Trial Performance." *Int J Sports Med* 36, no. 2 (2015): 107-12.

Levett, D.Z., et al. "The role of nitrogen oxides in human adaptation to hypoxia." *Sci Rep* 1 (2011): 109.

Li, H., et al. "Nitrate-reducing bacteria on rat tongues." *Appl Environ Microbiol* 63, no. 3 (1997): 924-30.

Lortie, M.J., et al. "Bioactive products of arginine in sepsis: tissue and plasma composition after LPS and iNOS blockade." *Am J Physiol Cell Physiol* 278, no. 6 (2000): C1191-9.

Luiking, Y.C., and N.E. Deutz. "Isotopic investigation of nitric oxide metabolism in disease." *Curr Opin Clin Nutr Metab Care* 6, no. 1 (2003): 103-8.

Lundberg, J.O., et al. "Cardioprotective effects of vegetables: is nitrate the answer?" *Nitric Oxide* 15, no. 4 (2006): 359-62.

Lundberg, J.O., et al. "Intragastric nitric oxide production in humans: measurements in expelled air." *Gut* 35, no. 11 (1994): 1543-6.

Lundberg, J.O., et al. "Nitrate, bacteria and human health." *Nat Rev Microbiol* 2, no. 7 (2004): 593-602.

Lundberg, J.O., E. Weitzberg, and M.T. Gladwin. "The nitrate-nitrite-nitric oxide pathway in physiology and therapeutics." *Nat Rev Drug Discov* 7, no. 8 (2008): 156-167.

McKnight, G.M., et al. "Chemical synthesis of nitric oxide in the stomach from dietary nitrate in humans." *Gut* 40, no. 2 (1997): 211-4.

McMahon, C.N., C.J. Smith, and R. Shabsigh. "Treating erectile dysfunction when PDE5 inhibitors fail." *BMJ* 332, no. 7541 (2006): 589-92.

Mensinga, T.T., G.J. Speijers, and J. Meulenbelt. "Health implications of exposure to environmental nitrogenous compounds." *Toxicol Rev* 22, no. 1 (2003): 41-51.

Moir, J.W.B., ed. *Nitrogen Cycling in Bacteria: Molecular Analysis.* Norfolk, UK: Caister Academic Press, 2011.

Nadtochiy, S.M., and E.K. Redman. "Mediterranean diet and cardioprotection: the role of nitrite, polyunsaturated fatty acids, and polyphenols." *Nutrition* 27, no. 7-8 (2011): 733-44.

Nagamani, S.C., et al. "Nitric-oxide supplementation for treatment of long-term complications in argininosuccinic aciduria." *Am J Hum Genet* 90, no. 5 (2012): 836-46.

Nunez de Gonzalez, M.T., et al. "A survey of nitrate and nitrite concentrations in conventional and organic-labeled raw vegetables at retail." *J Food Sci* 80, no. 5 (2015): C942-9.

Nunez de Gonzalez, M.T., et al. "Survey of residual nitrite and nitrate in conventional and organic/natural/uncured/indirectly cured meats available at retail in the United States." *J Agric Food Chem* 60, no. 15 (2012): 3981-90.

Ohta, N., et al. "Nitric oxide metabolites and adrenomedullin in human breast milk." *Early Hum Dev* 78, no. 1 (2004): 61-5.

Oldfield, E.H., et al. "Safety and pharmacokinetics of sodium nitrite in patients with subarachnoid hemorrhage: A Phase IIA study." *J Neurosurg* 119, no. 3 (2013): 634-41.

Pennington, J. "Dietary exposure models for nitrates and nitrites." *Food Control* 9, no. 6 (1998): 385-395.

Perros, F., et al. "Nebivolol for improving endothelial dysfunction, pulmonary vascular remodeling, and right heart function in pulmonary hypertension." *J Am Coll Cardiol* 65, no. 7 (2015): 668-80.

Petersson, J., et al. "Gastroprotective and blood pressure lowering effects of dietary nitrate are abolished by an antiseptic mouthwash." *Free Radic Biol Med* 46, no. 8 (2009): 1068-75.

Pie, J.E., et al. "Age-related decline of inducible nitric oxide synthase gene expression in primary cultured rat hepatocytes." *Mol Cells* 13, no. 3 (2002): 399-406.

Pinheiro, L.C., et al. "Gastric S-nitrosothiol formation drives the antihypertensive effects of oral sodium nitrite and nitrate in a rat model of renovascular hypertension." *Free Radic Biol Med* 87 (2015): 252-62.

Pinheiro, L.C., et al. "Increase in gastric pH reduces hypotensive effect of oral sodium nitrite in rats." *Free Radic Biol Med* 53, no. 4 (2012): 701-9.

Porst, H., et al. "Efficacy of tadalafil for the treatment of erectile dysfunction at 24 and 36 hours after dosing: a randomized controlled trial." *Urology* 62, no. 1 (2003): 121-5; discussion 125-6.

Qin, L., et al. "Sialin (SLC17A5) functions as a nitrate transporter in the plasma membrane." *Proc Natl Acad Sci USA* 109, no. 33 (2012): 13434-9.

Rahma, M., et al. "Effects of furosemide on the tubular reabsorption of nitrates in anesthetized dogs." *Eur J Pharmacol* 428, no. 1 (2001): 113-9.

Rassaf, T., et al. "Nitric oxide synthase-derived plasma nitrite predicts exercise capacity." *Br J Sports Med* 41, no. 10 (2007): 669-73; discussion 673.

Ross, R. "Atherosclerosis—an inflammatory disease." *N Engl J Med* 340, no. 2 (1999): 115-26.

Schulman, S.P., et al. "L-arginine therapy in acute myocardial infarction: the Vascular Interaction With Age in Myocardial Infarction (VINTAGE MI) randomized clinical trial." *JAMA* 295, no. 1 (2006): 58-64.

Sobko, T., et al. "Dietary nitrate in Japanese traditional foods lowers diastolic blood pressure in healthy volunteers." *Nitric Oxide* 22, no. 2 (2010): 136-40.

Soltis, E.E. "Effect of age on blood pressure and membrane-dependent vascular responses in the rat." *Circ Res* 61, no. 6 (1987): 889-97.

Spiegelhalder, B., G. Eisenbrand, and R. Preussmann. "Influence of dietary nitrate on nitrite content of human saliva: possible relevance to in vivo formation of N-nitroso compounds." *Food Cosmet Toxicol* 14, no. 6 (1976): 545-8.

Stamler, J.S., et al. "S-nitrosylation of proteins with nitric oxide: synthesis and characterization of biologically active compounds." *Proc Natl Acad Sci USA* 89 (1992): 444-448.

Taddei, S., et al. "Age-related reduction of NO availability and oxidative stress in humans." *Hypertension* 38, no. 2 (2001): 274-9.

Tang, Y., H. Garg, Y.J. Geng, and N.S. Bryan. "Nitric oxide bioactivity of traditional Chinese medicines used for cardiovascular indications." *Free Radic Biol Med* 47, no. 6 (2009): 835-40.

Tuso, P., S.R. Stoll, and W.W. Li. "A plant-based diet, atherogenesis, and coronary artery disease prevention." *Perm J* 19, no. 1 (2015): 62-7.

Van Der Loo, B., et al. "Enhanced peroxynitrite formation is associated with vascular aging." *J Exp Med* 192, no. 12 (2000): 1731-44.

Van Eijk, H.M., Y.C. Luiking, and N.E. Deutz. "Methods using stable isotopes to measure nitric oxide (NO) synthesis in the L-arginine/NO pathway in health and disease." *J Chromatogr B Analyt Technol Biomed Life Sci* 851, no. 1-2 (2007): 172-85.

Vanhatalo, A., et al. "Acute and chronic effects of dietary nitrate supplementation on blood pressure and the physiological responses to moderate-intensity and incremental exercise."

Am J Physiol Regul Integr Comp Physiol 299, no. 4 (2010): R1121-31.

Vita, J.A., et al. "Coronary vasomotor response to acetylcholine relates to risk factors for coronary artery disease." *Circulation* 81, no. 2 (1990): 491-7.

Walker, R. "The metabolism of dietary nitrites and nitrates." *Biochem Soc Trans* 24, no. 3 (1996): 780-5.

Wang, Y.R., G.C. Alexander, and R.S. Stafford. "Outpatient hypertension treatment, treatment intensification, and control in Western Europe and the United States." *Arch Intern Med* 167, no. 2 (2007): 141-7.

Webb, A.J., et al. "Acute blood pressure lowering, vasoprotective, and antiplatelet properties of dietary nitrate via bioconversion to nitrite." *Hypertension* 51, no. 3 (2008): 784-90.

Weimann, J., et al. "Sildenafil is a pulmonary vasodilator in awake lambs with acute pulmonary hypertension." *Anesthesiology* 92, no. 6 (2000): 1702-12.

Wennmalm, A., et al. "Metabolism and excretion of nitric oxide in humans. An experimental and clinical study." *Circ Res* 73, no. 6 (1993): 1121-7.

Wilson, A.M., et al. "L-arginine supplementation in peripheral arterial disease: no benefit and possible harm." *Circulation* 116, no. 2 (2007): 188-95.

Wright, J.T., Jr., et al. "A Randomized Trial of Intensive versus Standard Blood-Pressure Control." *N Engl J Med* 373, no. 22 (2015): 2103-16.

Yazji, I., et al. "Endothelial TLR4 activation impairs intestinal microcirculatory perfusion in necrotizing enterocolitis via eNOS-NO-nitrite signaling." *Proc Natl Acad Sci USA* 110, no. 23 (2013): 9451-6.

Zand, J., F. Lanza, H.K. Garg, and N.S. Bryan. "All-natural nitrite and nitrate containing dietary supplement promotes nitric oxide production and reduces triglycerides in humans." Nutr Res 31, no. 4 (2011): 262-9.

Zhou, X.J., et al. "Association of renal injury with nitric oxide deficiency in aged SHR: prevention by hypertension control with AT1 blockade." Kidney Int 62, no. 3 (2002): 914-21.

Resources

www.drnathansbryan.com

www.functionalnitricoxidenutrition.com

www.nitricoxidesociety.org

www.ingramcontent.com/pod-product-compliance
Lightning Source LLC
Chambersburg PA
CBHW060910280326
41934CB00007B/1262